PARASITIC WORMS

# The Wykeham Science Series

*General Editors:*

PROFESSOR SIR NEVILL MOTT, F.R.S.
Emeritus Cavendish Professor of Physics
University of Cambridge

G. R. NOAKES
Formerly Senior Physics Master
Uppingham School

*Biology Editor:*

W. B. YAPP
Formerly Senior Lecturer
University of Birmingham

*The Authors:*

D. W. T. CROMPTON graduated from the University of Cambridge, and is now Lecturer in Parasitology there. He also holds an adjunct appointment in nutritional sciences at Cornell University, and is an editor of the journal *Parasitology*.

S. M. JOYNER has carried out research in zoology and parasitology at the University of Cambridge, and taught biology at Blyth Jex School, Norwich. She is now chief examiner for A-level biology project work for the Cambridge Examination Board.

# PARASITIC WORMS

**D. W. T. CROMPTON**
*University of Cambridge*

and

**S. M. JOYNER**
*Formerly Blyth Jex School, Norwich*

ALERE FLAMMAM

WYKEHAM PUBLICATIONS (LONDON) LTD
(A member of the Taylor & Francis Group)
1980

First published 1980 by Wykeham Publications (London) Ltd.



Printed in Great Britain by
Biddles Ltd, Guildford, Surrey

**British Library Cataloguing in Publication Data**

Crompton, D W T
Parasitic worms. – (The Wykeham science series; 57).
1. Worms, Intestinal and parasitic
I. Title II. Joyner, S M
595'.1'04524 QL392

ISBN 0-85109-830-4

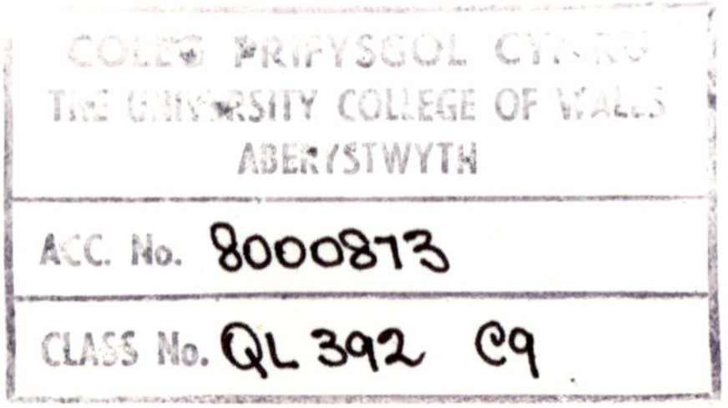

# Contents

# Acknowledgements

We are grateful to the following colleagues who have read various drafts either of the whole book or of sections of it: Mrs E. M. Crompton, Hinchingbrooke School; Dr P. J. F. Henderson, Department of Biochemistry, University of Cambridge; Dr A. M. Lackie, Department of Zoology, University of Glasgow; Miss C. A. Lockwood, University of Birmingham; Dr J. Martin, The Molteno Institute, University of Cambridge; Dr E. A. Munn, A.R.C. Institute of Animal Physiology; Mrs P. Munn, The Perse School for Girls; Dr V. R. Parshad, Punjab Agricultural University; Miss G. Stock, Hinchingbrooke School; Dr J. N. Thomas, Department of Biology, The Open University. We also thank Dr S. Conway Morris, Dr D. Franks and Dr R. A. Klein for helpful discussions. We have gladly incorporated many of their suggestions into the text and wish to point out that they are in no way responsible for the errors that remain.

We thank Dr E. A. Munn for providing the electron micrographs which make up figs. 6.4, 6.5, 6.6 and 6.7; Professor L. T. Threadgold, Department of Zoology, The Queen's University, Belfast, for those which form figs. 1.11, 1.33 and 1.35; and Dr D. A. Halton, Department of Zoology, The Queen's University, Belfast, for the photomicrograph used for fig. 7.10. Some of the figures and tables are original and some are direct reproductions from the published works of other authors. The majority of the figures have been redrawn and variously adapted from many sources and acknowledgement to the authors concerned has been made in the text. The citation of an article or book in a figure legend or table title usually indicates that relatively little change has been made during the preparation of our illustration. Consequently, we thank the following copyright owners for permission to use their materials: Academic Press Inc. (London) Ltd for table 3.4 and figs. 1.10, 1.36, 1.56, 1.57, 1.59, 4.1, 7.18, 7.26, 8.8, 8.17 and 8.20; *Acta Parasitologica Polonica* for fig. 3.5; Addison-Wesley Publishing Company for fig. 10.1; American Institute of Biological Sciences for fig. 7.1; American Microscopical Society for figs. 3.42 and 7.7; American Society of Parasitologists for figs. 1.16, 1.17, 1.28, 1.37, 1.38, 1.39, 3.10, 3.22, 3.38, 3.40, 3.41, 5.6, 7.27, 8.18 and 8.19; American Society of Tropical Medicine and Hygiene for fig. 10.2; Appleton-Century-Crofts for figs. 3.18 and 3.27; Australian Society for Parasitology and Pergamon Press Ltd for fig 7.10; Blackwell Scientific Publications for fig. 1.58; Cambridge University Press for figs. 1.5, 1.6, 1.7, 1.8, 1.12, 1.14, 1.29, 1.30, 1.31, 1.42, 1.43, 1.45, 2.6, 2.7, 2.8, 3.8, 3.9, 3.19, 3.21, 3.23, 3.26, 3.29, 3.30, 3.32, 3.36, 3.37, 3.45, 3.46, 3.47, 3.48, 3.49, 4.2, 4.4, 4.5, 5.3, 5.4, 5.5, 6.3, 7.20, 7.24, 7.29, 7.30, 8.1, 8.2, 8.10, 8.11, 8.12, 8.13, 8.14 and 9.3; Company of Biologists Ltd for fig. 7.23; B. G. and M. B. Chitwood for fig. 3.16; W. H. Freeman and B. Bracegirdle for figs. 1.3, 1.26, 1.32 and 3.33; S. Karger AG for fig. 7.11; Lea and Febiger for fig. 3.43; Macmillan Journals Ltd for fig. 4.3; McGraw-Hill Book Company for figs. 1.41, 1.44, 1.51, 1.53, 1.55, 1.60 and 3.34; Mrs J. A. McNeill for fig. 7.8; Marine Biological Association of the UK for fig. 5.1; Marine Biology Laboratory (Woods Hole) for fig. 1.15; R. Muller for fig. 7.6; National Research Council of Canada for fig. 5.2; *Norwegian Journal of Zoology* for table 4.3 and fig. 1.25; Penguin Books Ltd for fig. 7.25; Rockefeller University Press for fig. 7.21; The Royal Society for figs. 1.18, 1.19, 1.20, 1.21, 1.22, 1.23 and 1.24; The Royal Swedish Academy of Sciences for fig. 7.4; W. B. Saunders Company for figs. 9.5, 9.6, 9.7, 9.8 and 9.12; Society for Experimental Biology for fig. 9.4; Springer-Verlag for fig. 1.2; J. D. Smyth for fig. 8.9; US Government Printing Office for fig. 7.9; University of Illinois Press for fig. 3.20; University of Minnesota Press for figs. 3.31 and 3.35; University of Toronto Press for figs. 1.14 and 3.17; John Wiley and Sons Inc. for fig. 7.5; Wistar Institute Press for fig. 3.15; World Health Organization for table 10.2; Zoological Institute of Uppsala for fig. 7.17; *Zoologica Poloniae* for fig. 7.19.

Finally we thank Miss Catharine Frattasi for her careful preparation of the typescript.

D. W. T. CROMPTON and S. M. JOYNER
November 1978

# Preface

Asa Chandler, one of the founding fathers of parasitology, once stated that the name 'worm' is an indefinite though suggestive term popularly applied to any elongated creeping thing that is not obviously something else. Parasitic worms from animal hosts are often called helminths, and in this book we have used the terms 'worm' and 'helminth' freely and interchangeably for both ectoparasitic and endoparasitic species. We have taken ectoparasitic worms to be those living where they can be seen with little or no dissection of the host. Endoparasitic worms have been assumed to be those living out of sight in the organs, cavities and tissues of the host. We have avoided the semantic debate about whether the lumina of the alimentary, respiratory and urinogenital tracts are inside or outside the body; worms which live in such places are assumed to be endoparasites.

This book is intended to introduce, to students with or without previous knowledge of parasitology, certain aspects of the biology of parasitic worms and some of the features of parasitism. Many generalizations have been made and these should be accepted with caution since exceptions can invariably be found. The glossary at the end of the book provides explanations for some of the biological terms which have not been defined in the text. Our intention has been to allow the figures to take the place of detailed descriptions of morphology. Where appropriate, as in the case of an illustration of the structure of a particular species, a scale bar has been included, but scales have not always been added to diagrams such as those intended to aid in the interpretation of electron micrographs.

The scientific names of parasitic worms are complicated and sometimes difficult to remember. Seven species (*Polystoma integerrimum, Fasciola hepatica, Schistosoma mansoni, Hymenolepis diminuta, Moniliformis dubius, Nippostrongylus brasiliensis* and *Ascaris lumbricoides*) have been cited quite frequently and so have usually been referred to by their generic names only. *Ascaris*, which has been investigated intensively, presents a special problem because most

authorities now recognize *A. lumbricoides* from man and *A. suum* from pigs as separate species. We have retained the single name, but have sometimes indicated the animal from which the worm was obtained.

Helminths have been studied for a long time. Over a hundred years ago, Spencer Cobbold wrote: 'The happiest, and perhaps after all, the most truly philosophic way of studying the entozoa (parasitic worms) is to regard them as a peculiar fauna, destined to occupy a peculiar territory. That territory is the widespread domain of the bodies of man and animals. Each animal or host may be regarded as a continent and each part or viscus of his body may be noted as a district. Each district has its special attractions for particular parasitic forms; yet at the same time, neither the district nor the continent are suitable localities as a permanent resting-place for the invader. None of the internal parasites "continue in one stay"; all have a tendency to roam; migration is the very soul of their prosperity; change of residence the *sine qua non* of their existence, whilst a blockade in the interior, prolonged beyond the proper period, terminates only in cretification and death'.

NOW READ ON . . .

# 1. Introduction to the worms

Parasitism is a dynamic relationship between living organisms in which all the energy and nutrients needed by both partners are obtained by the host. In many cases, a delicate physiological equilibrium develops between the activity of the parasite and the resistance of the host, and signs of the association may be difficult to detect. Unfortunately, there are some host–parasite relationships in which the equilibrium tilts away from the host so that the signs, symptoms and consequences of disease become apparent. Millions of people and animals and acres of crops are afflicted and depressed by parasitic infections. The contribution of parasitic worms, especially the blood flukes, hookworms and filarial worms, to this picture of silent suffering is vast and the economic implications are enormous. It is hardly surprising that helminths are often viewed with disgust and revulsion. While agreeing unreservedly that every effort must be made to relieve mankind from the burden of parasitic disease, the zoologist cannot help but marvel at the adaptations of parasitic worms and the intricacy of host–parasite relationships.

Although there exists a variety of unusual animals which have adopted the parasitic habit and are worm-like in appearance, the overwhelming majority of parasitic worms from all regions of the earth belong to the phyla Platyhelminthes (flatworms), Acanthocephala (spiny-headed worms) and Aschelminthes (including the roundworms). A classification of these animals is given in table 1.1 and a diagram showing the phylogenetic relationships of the parasites and their hosts is shown in fig. 1.1. Schemes of classification aim to set out the natural relationships between organisms, but this ideal is rarely achieved. Each taxonomist is likely to have convincing evidence supporting his or her own scheme and the one in table 1.1 is for convenience rather than for completeness. Good reasons can be advanced for dropping the term 'Trematoda' from the platyhelminths. On the other hand, use of the word 'trematode' to mean parasitic fluke is well established and is likely to remain for a long time.

TABLE 1.1. *A traditional classification of the chief groups of animal parasitic worms.*

Phylum. PLATYHELMINTHES (flatworms)

- Class. TREMATODA (flukes)
  - Order. Monogenea (*Polystoma*)
  - Order. Aspidogastrea
  - Order. Digenea
    - Sub-order. Gasterostomata (1 family)
    - Sub-order. Prostomata (46 families; *Fasciola* and *Schistosoma*)
- Class. CESTODA
  - Sub-class. Cestodaria
    - Order. Amphilinidea
    - Order. Gyrocotylidea
  - Sub-class. Eucestoda (tapeworms)
    - Order. Tetraphyllidea
    - Order. Trypanorhyncha
    - Order. Pseudophyllidea
    - Order. Cyclophyllidea (*Hymenolepis*)

Phylum. ACANTHOCEPHALA (spiny-headed worms)

- Order. Palaeacanthocephala
- Order. Archiacanthocephala (*Moniliformis*)
- Order. Eoacanthocephala

Phylum. ASCHELMINTHES

- Class. NEMATODA (roundworms)
  - Sub-class. Aphasmida
    - Order. Trichinellida
    - Order. Dioctophymatida
  - Sub-class. Phasmida
    - Order. Rhabditida
    - Order. Strongylida
      - Sub-order. Strongylina (*Nippostrongylus*)
      - Sub-order. Trichostrongylina
      - Sub-order. Metastrongylina
    - Order. Ascarida
      - Sub-order. Ascaridina (*Ascaris*)
      - Sub-order. Oxyurina
      - Sub-order. Heterakina
    - Order. Spirurida
      - Sub-order. Spirurina
      - Sub-order. Camallanina
      - Sub-order. Filariina

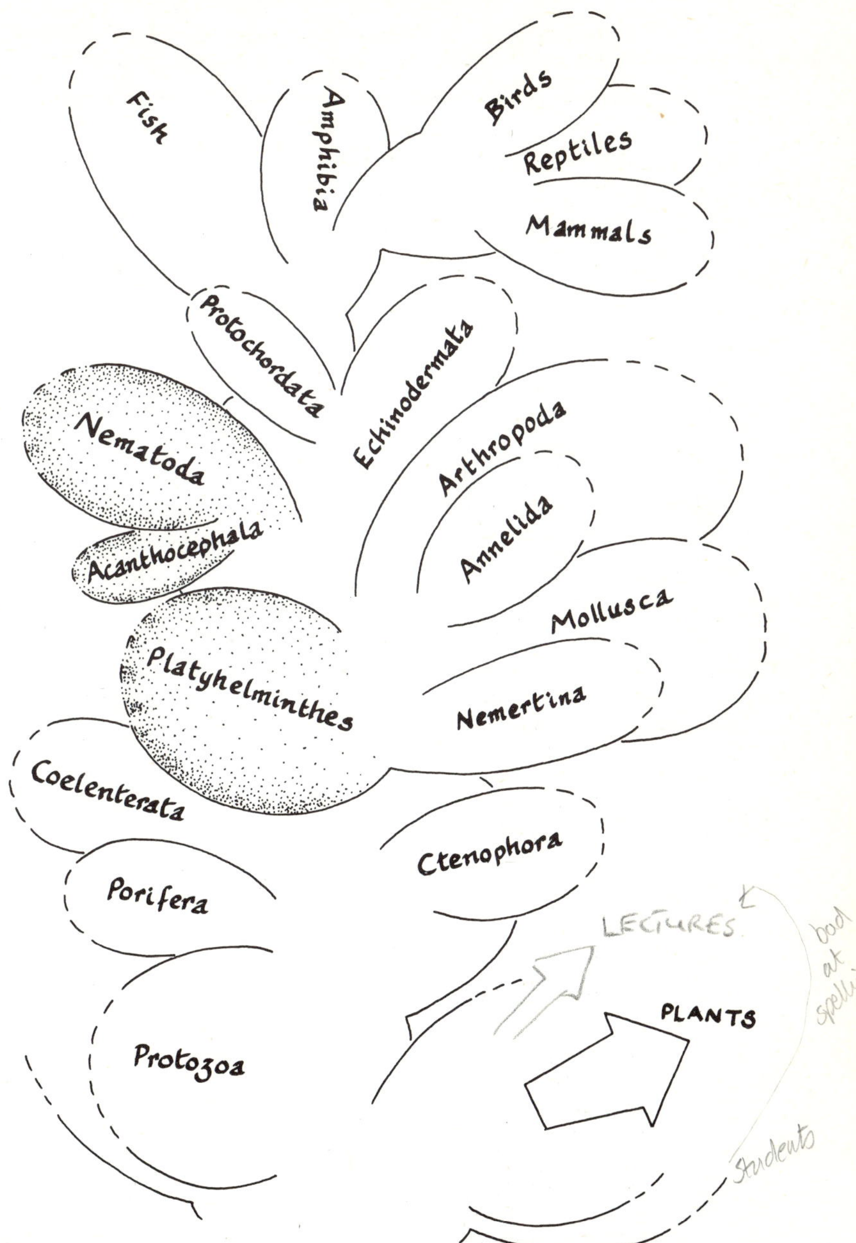


Fig. 1.1. A diagrammatic representation of one view of suspected phylogenetic relationships in the animal kingdom. Stippling indicates the main groups of parasitic worms.

Despite the obvious morphological similarities between adult monogeneans and digeneans (see below), recent comparative investigations of the development of the different groups of platyhelminths have indicated that monogeneans may be more closely related to cestodes than to digeneans. Some experts advocate that, in order to avoid implying a fairly close relationship between monogeneans and digeneans, both groups should be given the status of class rather than order within the phylum (table 1.1). This rather academic point illustrates how schemes of classification are in a constant state of flux if the animals they deal with are exciting and stimulating to study.

There is very little information about the origin of parasitic worms. Parasitism probably evolved as a feature of life long before the existence of vertebrates, when an extraordinary invertebrate fauna flourished in the seas at least 600 million years ago. Maybe the association began when animals shared the same burrow or shared the same food. Perhaps one type of animal became a predator on another and perhaps its occasional failure to digest the prey led to the survival of the prey within its captor. Perhaps one smaller species tended to bore into the rotting corpses of larger species and perhaps the urge to enter living bodies soon followed. Many other speculative suggestions could be made about the evolution of host–helminth relationships.

## 1.1. *Platyhelminthes—flukes and tapeworms*

Platyhelminths are generally flattened in the dorso-ventral plane with an obvious and specialized anterior end. They have no body cavity, and neither a circulatory system nor a respiratory system; their excretory system is characterized by the presence of flame cells. The adult body is bounded by a continuous tegument of living cytoplasm; there is little evidence of a toughened and inert cuticle. Circular, longitudinal and diagonal muscles make up part of the tissues. The worms are usually hermaphrodites with complex reproductive apparatus. In addition to the Monogenea, Digenea and Cestoda, in which all the known species are parasites, there is a third group called the Turbellaria. Most turbellarians are free-living, but there are some exceptions. For example, *Fecampia erythrocephala* is a small turbellarian about 12 mm long which lives in the body of common shore crabs. The mature worms leave their hosts and settle on the undersurfaces of boulders near the low-water mark. Here they secrete a white, rubbery cocoon around themselves, lay their eggs and die. Eventually, small larval stages develop from the eggs, leave the shelter of the cocoon and are assumed to penetrate the cuticle of the appropriate species of crab.

Most species of parasitic flatworm are flukes belonging to the Monogenea and Digenea (table 1.1). Flukes usually have creamy coloured, semitransparent, leaf-shaped bodies and the adult stages possess muscular suckers and holdfast organs, an alimentary tract with a mouth but no anus, and the other features of the platyhelminths already described. The notion that food is sucked in by the suckers is erroneous. Various aspects of the morphology of mature monogeneans, aspidogastreans and digeneans are illustrated in figs. 1.2–1.15. When identification is being attempted, it should be remembered that the development, behaviour and host specificity of a helminth are often as important as its morphology.

Aspidogastreans are distinguished from other flukes by the possession of a prominent adhesive disc (fig. 1.2) and an array of sensory marginal organs. They appear to be associated with marine and freshwater hosts. Some species mature in the bodies of bivalves, others amongst the gills of snails and others, like *Aspidogaster limacoides*, inhabit the alimentary tract of fish. It is just possible, therefore, that the host–parasite relationships of aspidogastreans provide a tentative basis for postulating that some of the parasites of vertebrates were acquired as their ancestors fed on the well-established invertebrate fauna.

Most monogenean flukes are ectoparasitic on the gills and skin of fishes, although some species have become adapted for an endoparasitic existence in some unusual locations. The adult *Polystoma* (fig. 1.3) inhabits the bladders of frogs and toads, but the immature forms begin the host–parasite relationship on the gills of the tadpole. *Calicotyle kroeri* lives in the cloaca of rays and *Oculotrema hippopotami* under the eyelids of the hippopotamus. *Amphibdella flavolineata* is another extraordinary monogenean which flourishes for a time in the blood system of electric rays before invading the gills, where it leads an ectoparasitic life. Adult monogeneans are recognized morphologically by their well-developed posterior organs of attachment (fig. 1.4), which consist of suckers and hooks.

In contrast to monogenean flukes, the majority of digeneans are endoparasites, although adult members of the family Transversotrematidae are a notable exception. Most mature digeneans are relatively small in length. They possess two simple muscular suckers and the body is not infrequently armed with spines (figs. 1.6–1.8). In many species, the mouth is situated in the middle of the anterior or oral sucker (fig. 1.6), but in one group, the Gasterostomata (table

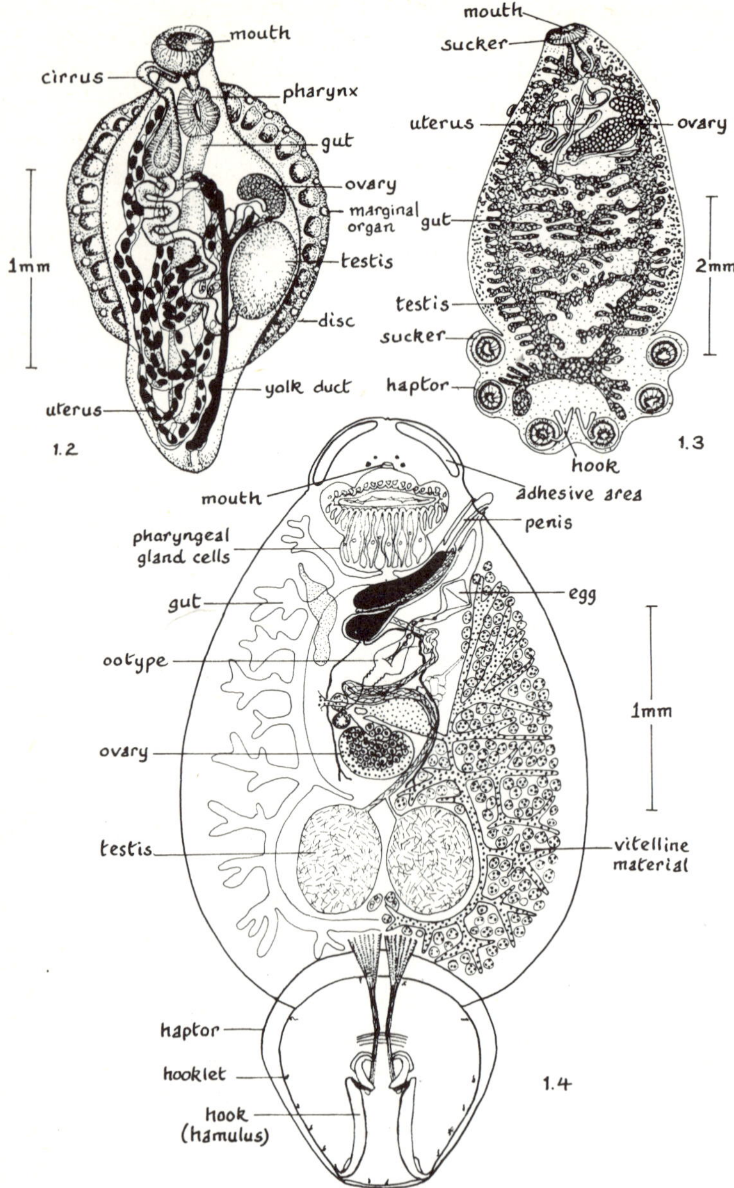


Figs. 1.2–1.4. Aspects of the morphology of mature aspidogastrean and monogenean flukes. 1.2 *Aspidogaster limacoides* (after Bychowsky and Bychowsky, 1934, *Z. Parasitenke*, 7, 125). 1.3. *Polystoma* sp. (after Freeman and Bracegirdle, 1971, *An Atlas of Invertebrate Structure*). 1.4. Ventral view of *Entobdella soleae* (after Kearn, 1971, In: *Ecology and Physiology of Parasites*).

1.1), the mouth is located much nearer to the middle of the body (fig. 1.12). There are also notable exceptions to the generalization that digeneans are hermaphrodites. The schistosomes or blood flukes are dioecious and the adults live in pairs in the blood vessels of their hosts (fig. 1.13). Flukes of the family Didymozoidae, which are cyst-dwellers in the tissues of fish, have several unusual features associated with reproduction. For example, individuals of *Kollikeria filicollis* appear to function as separate males and females, but the females possess small testes and the males have female features (fig. 1.14). *Allocreadium alloneotenicum* is a typical digenean in that it is a hermaphrodite, but the need for a vertebrate host has been lost and reproduction is achieved in the body cavities of caddis fly larvae (fig. 1.15).

Although most members of the class Cestoda are true tapeworms, some anomalous species have been classified as the Cestodaria (table 1.1). Mature cestodarians are unsegmented hermaphrodites with a characteristic attachment organ and no alimentary tract. The amphilinids are generally found in the body cavities of fish, while the gyrocotylids, which have a specialized holdfast, called the funnel or rosette (fig. 1.16), usually live in the intestine of rat fish. True tapeworms (figs. 1.17 - 1.36), like cestodarians, have no alimentary tract at any stage of their life cycle. Food is absorbed through the body surface, which is now known in some respects to resemble the absorptive surface of the vertebrate intestine (figs. 1.33, 1.34, 1.36). This ultrastructural resemblance provides an interesting example of convergent evolution in which tissues of widely different origin appear to have become modified to perform the same task in the same manner.

In the majority of tapeworms (figs. 1.17–1.29), the flattened body shows three more or less clearly defined regions. The attachment organ at the anterior end is known as the scolex, and is usually equipped with suckers, hooks and well-developed musculature (figs. 1.29–1.31). Next follows the neck, which is the region where the segments or proglottides are generated, and the third region is the chain of clearly defined proglottides which makes up the bulk of the body or strobila (figs. 1.18–1.24). Very rarely several 'tapes' extend from one attachment organ, as in the case of *Cathetocephalus thatcheri* from a shark (fig. 1.17). A few tapeworms are famous for the length of their bodies. *Diphyllobothrium latum* may be 9 metres long with about 4000 proglottides. *Echinococcus granulosus*, on the other hand, is small enough to nestle between the villi of the small intestine of its host (fig. 1.26). In tapeworms, each proglottis usually contains

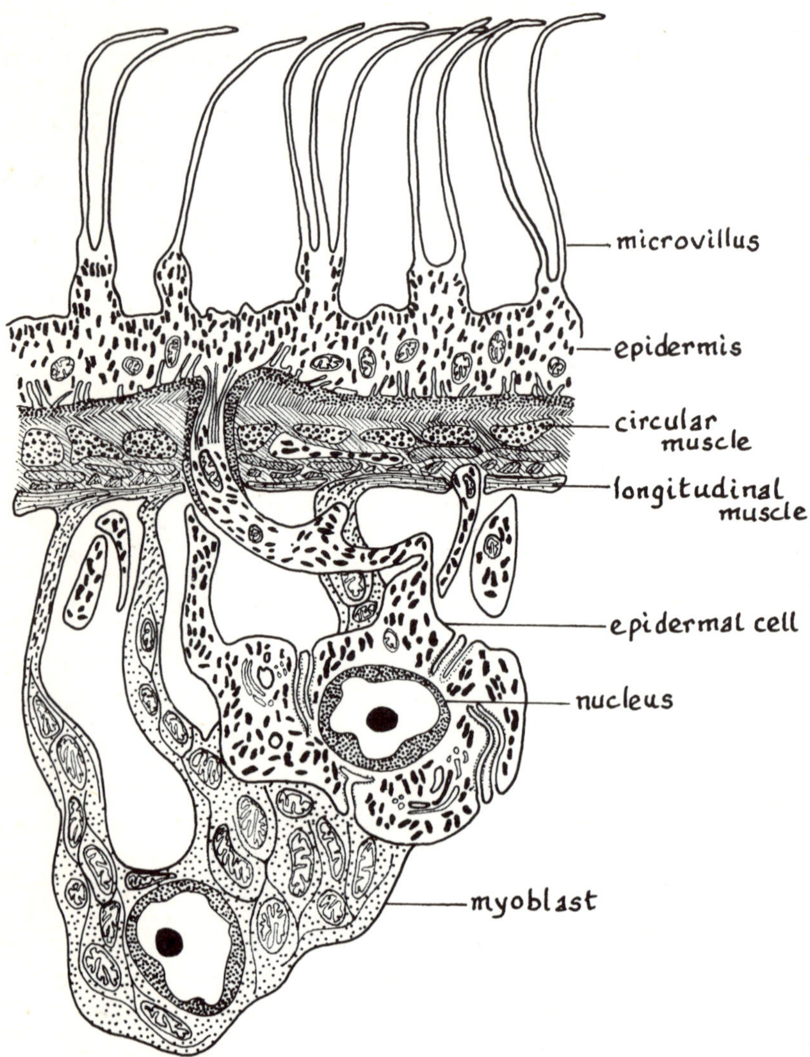


Fig. 1.5. Diagrammatic reconstruction, based on electron micrographs, of a longitudinal section through the dorsal body wall of *Entobdella soleae* (Monogenea) (after Lyons, 1970, *Parasitology*, **60**, 39).

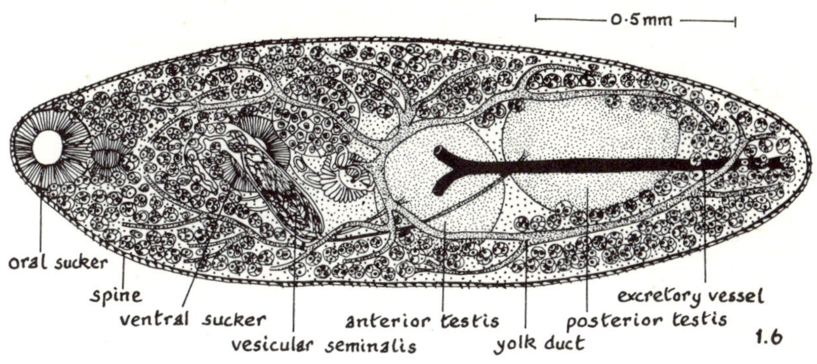


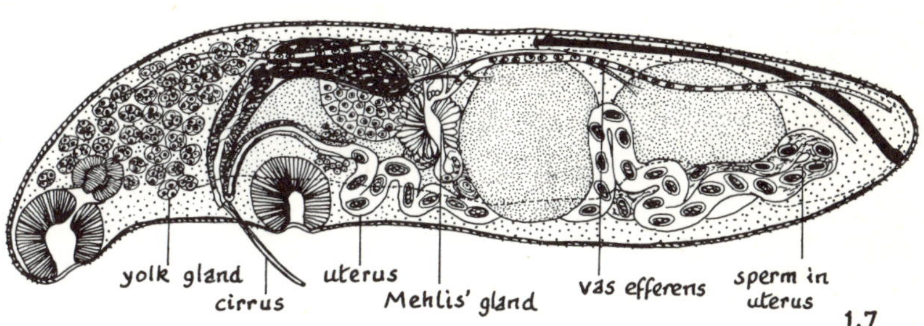


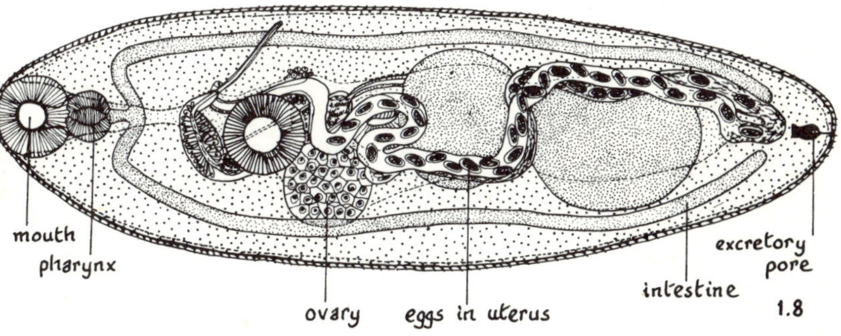


Figs. 1.6–1.8. Features of the morphology of adult *Plagiorchis megalorchis* (Digenea) from the domestic turkey (after Rees, 1952, *Parasitology*, **42**, 92). 1.6. Dorsal view. 1.7. Lateral view. 1.8. Ventral view.

male and female reproductive organs (figs. 1.22–1.24). The male system often matures before the female, but both sets of organs have become functional by the time the proglottides have reached the posterior part of the strobila. The eggs, which are found in the oldest proglottides, are shed when the proglottides become detached from the tape. The free proglottides may behave in one of three ways. In some species apolysis occurs, that is, the proglottis rots to expose the fully-developed eggs to the next host. In others there is euapolysis, that is, the detached gravid proglottis exists independently of the strobila for some time before the eggs are discharged. In still other

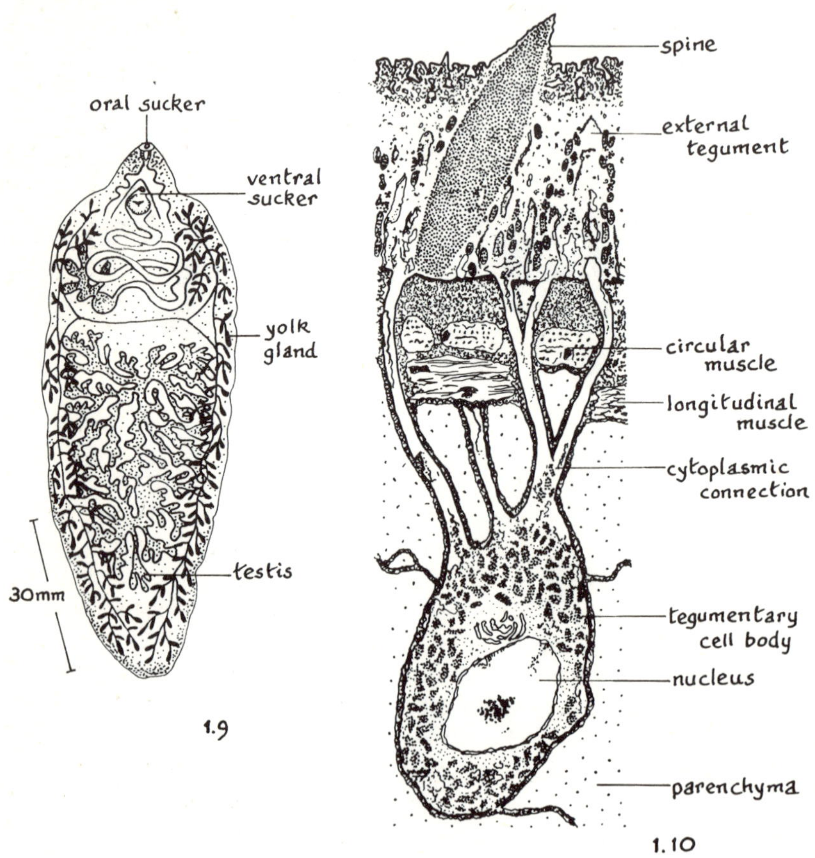


Figs. 1.9 and 1.10. Features of the morphology of adult *Fasciola hepatica* (Digenea, Prostomata, table 1.1). 1.9. General view. 1.10. Diagrammatic reconstruction, based on electron micrographs, of the structure of the body surface of *Fasciola* (after Lee, 1966, *Adv. Parasit.*, **4**, 187).

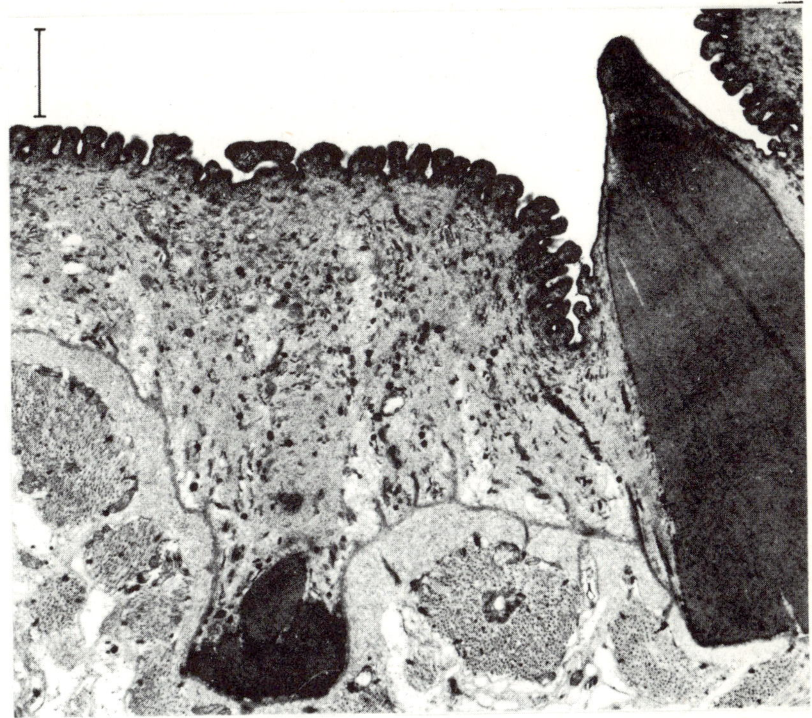

Fig. 1.11. Transmission electron micrograph of the tegument of the oral cone region of *Fasciola hepatica* (Digenea). The scale represents approximately 2 $\mu$m. (gift of L. T. Threadgold).

species hyperapolysis occurs, that is, the detached proglottis bears immature eggs whose development has to be completed before the proglottis dies. These itinerant proglottides can be a hazard to the unwary parasitologist, who may be deceived into assuming that he has found a new species of fluke.

Some members of the Eucestoda (table 1.1), however, cannot be considered as true tapeworms because their bodies do not consist of chains of proglottides. The family of the Pseudophyllidea (table 1.1) called the Caryophyllaeidae is very interesting in this respect because each worm has one set of reproductive organs and the body is unsegmented. *Archigetes sieboldi* (fig. 1.28) is a tiny caryophyllaeid which appears to have become neotenous; it matures in the body cavities of annelid worms and a vertebrate host is unnecessary. The genus *Dioecocestus* of the order Cyclophyllidea (table 1.1) includes, as its name indicates, tapeworms in which separate males and females are found.

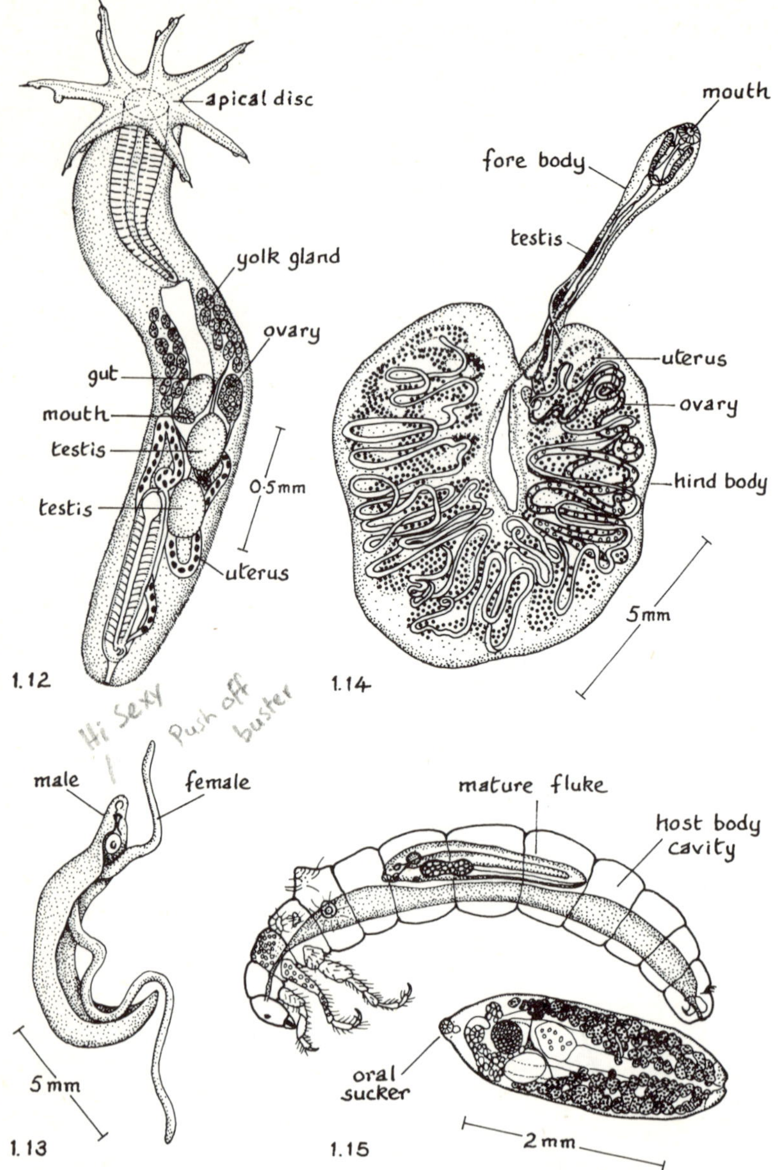


Fig. 1.12–1.15. Features of various mature Digenea. 1.12. *Alcicornis carangis* (Gasterostomata, table 1.1.) (after Rees, 1970, *Parasitology*, **60**, 195). 1.13. *Schistosoma mansoni;* the broad male supports the longer female in the gynaecophoric canal. 1.14. *Köllikeria filicollis*, a cyst-dwelling fluke (after Williams, 1959, *Parasitology*, **49**, 39). 1.15. *Allocreadium alloneotenicum* in the body cavity of a larval caddis fly (after Wootton, 1957, *Biol. Bull.* **113**, 302).

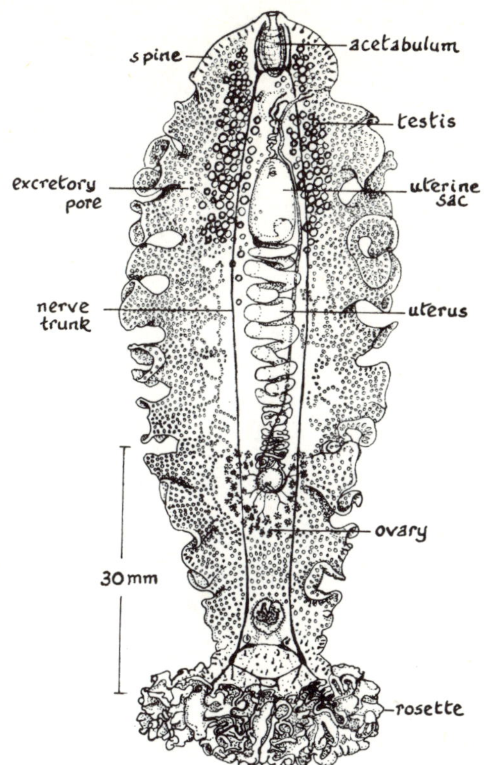


Fig. 1.16. The cestodarian *Gyrocotyle fimbriata* (after Lynch, 1945, *J. Parasit*, **31**, 418).

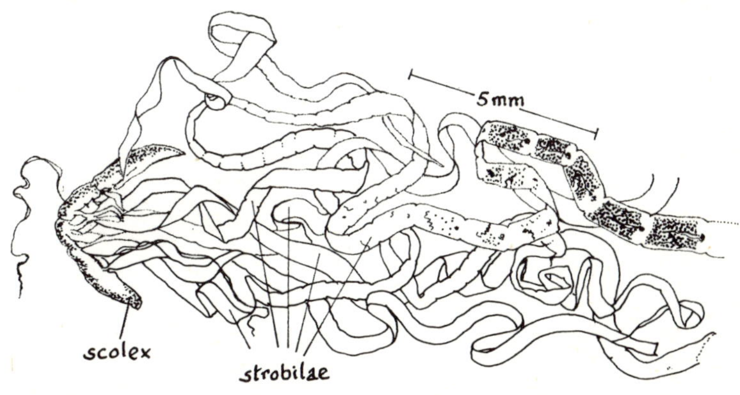


Fig. 1.17. *Cathetocephalus thatcheri*, a multistrobilate cestode (after Dailey and Overstreet, 1973, *J. Parasit.*, **59**, 469).

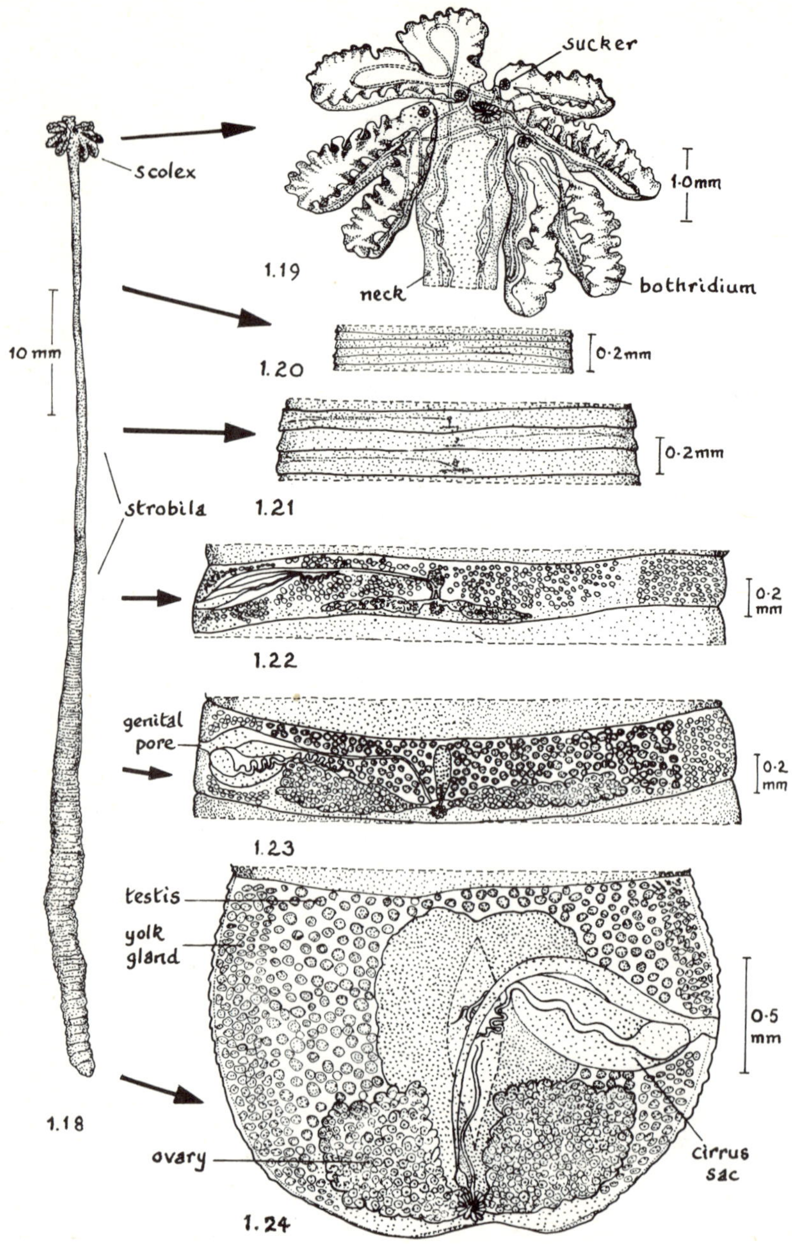


Figs. 1.18–1.24. The morphology of the cestode *Phyllobothrium lactuca* (after Williams, 1968, *Phil. Trans. Roy. Soc.* B, **253**, 231).

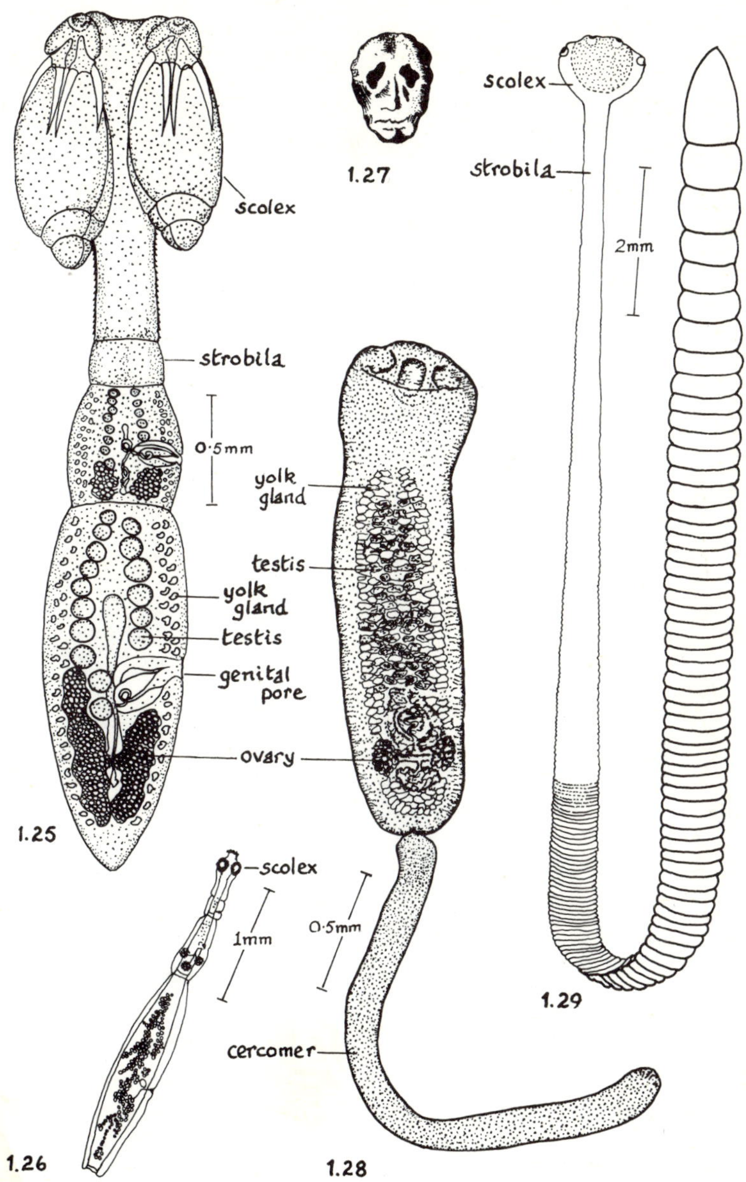


Figs. 1.25–1.29. Features of various mature Cestoda. 1.25. *Acanthobothrium tripartitum* (after Williams, 1969, *Nor. J. Zool.*, **17**, 1). 1.26 *Echinococcus granulosus* (after Freeman and Bracegirdle, 1971, *An Atlas of Invertebrate Structure*). 1.27. An early drawing of a tapeworm's head. 1.28. Mature *Archigetes sieboldi* from an aquatic annelid worm (after Calentine and Delong, 1966, *J. Parasit.*, **52**, 428). 1.29. *Discobothrium fallax* (after Williams, 1966, *Parasitology*, **56**, 227).

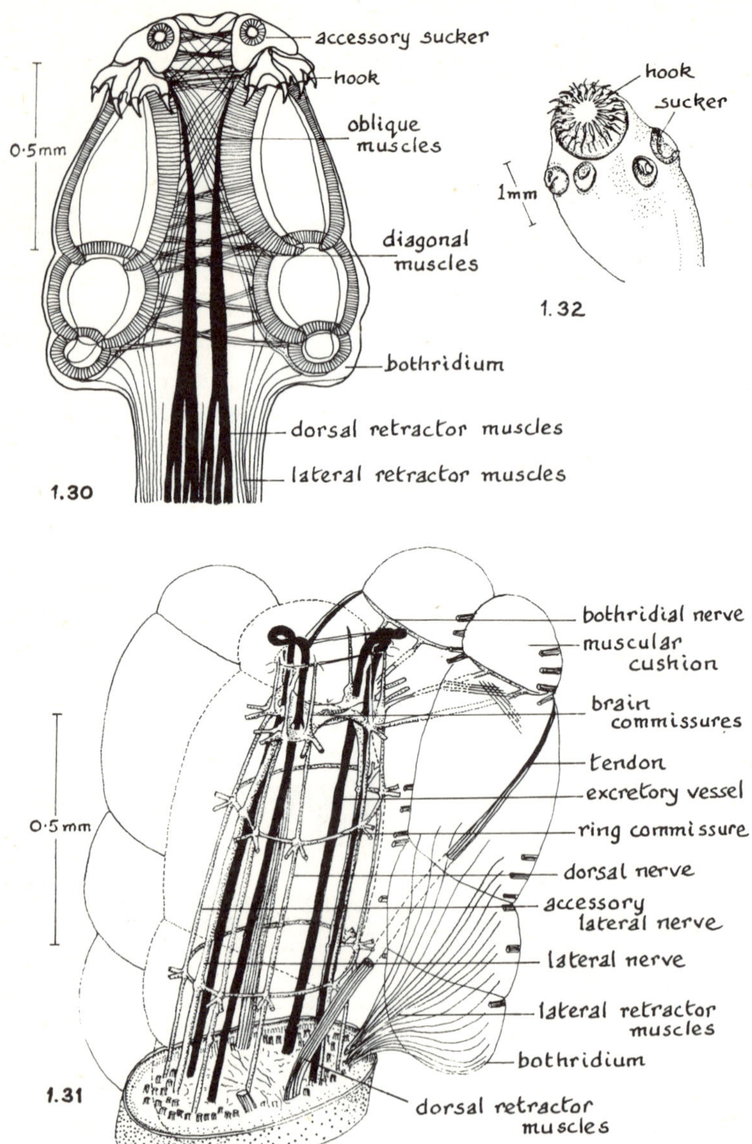


Figs. 1.30–1.32. Aspects of the structure of the cestode scolex. 1.30. Musculature in the scolex of *Acanthobothrium coronatum* (after Rees and Williams, 1965, *Parasitology*, **55**, 617). 1.31. Nervous and excretory systems in the scolex of *A. coronatum* (after Rees and Williams, 1965, *Parasitology*, **55**, 617). 1.32. Scolex of *Taenia* sp. (after Freeman and Bracegirdle, 1971, *An Atlas of Invertebrate Structure*).

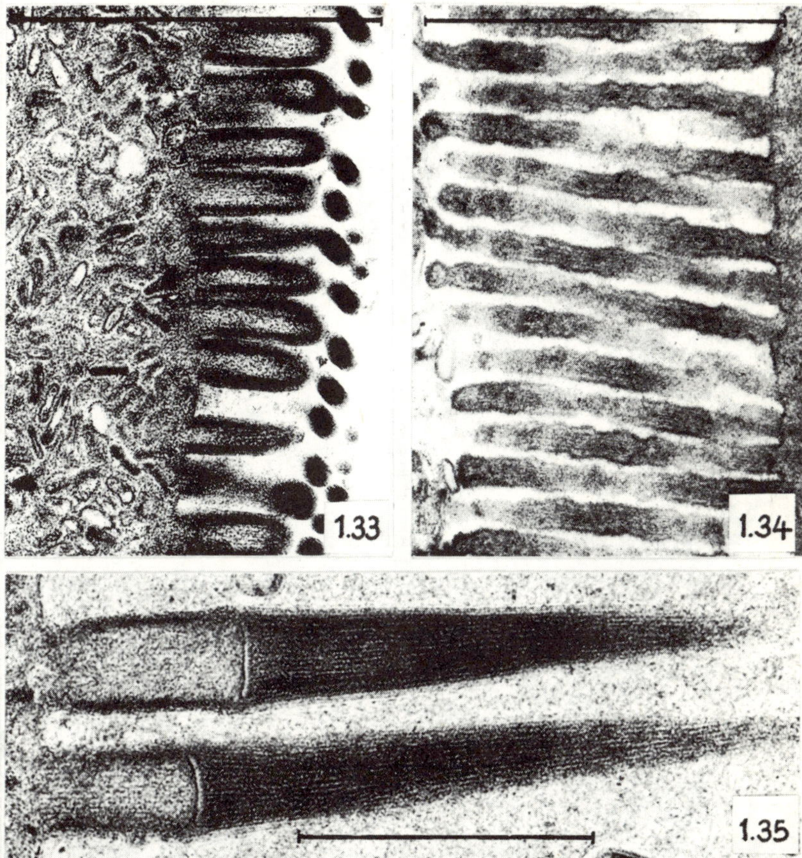


Figs. 1.33–1.35. Transmission electron micrographs. The scale represents approximately 1 $\mu$m. 1.33. Surface layers of adult *Hymenolepis diminuta* (Cestoda) (gift of L. T. Threadgold). 1.34. Microvilli at the surface of an epithelial cell from the small intestine of a rat. 1.35. Surface microtriches (microvilli) of a plerocercoid of *Schistocephalus solidus* (Cestoda) (gift of L. T. Threadgold).

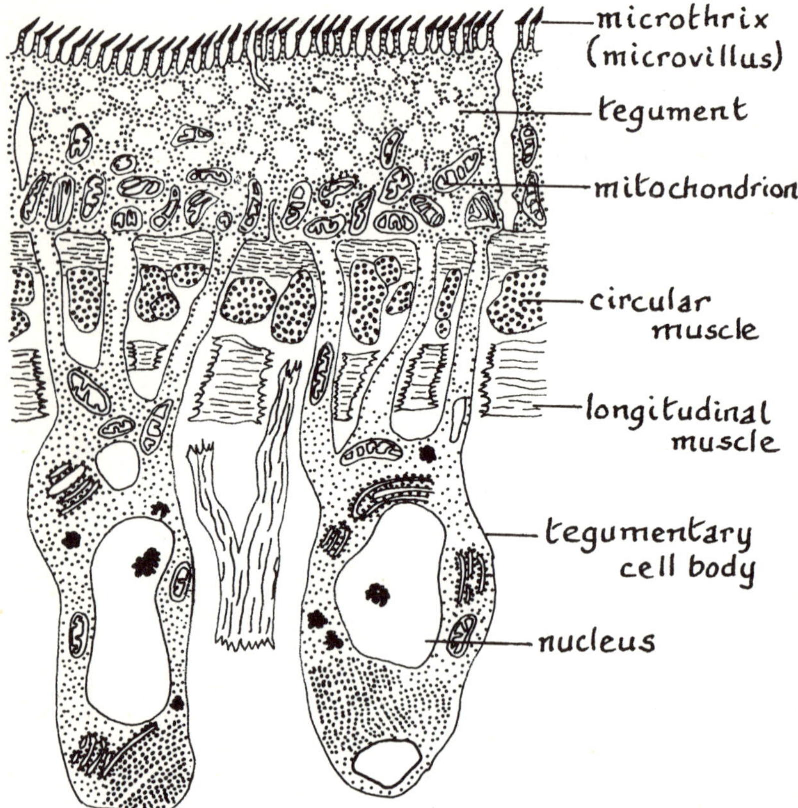


Fig. 1.36. Diagrammatic reconstruction, based on electron micrographs, of the structure of the tegument or surface tissue of *Dipylidium caninum* (Cestoda) (after Lee, 1966, *Adv. Parasit.*, **4**, 187).

## 1.2. *Acanthocephala—spiny-headed worms*

Acanthocephalan worms were not generally recognized as a separate group of animals until the middle of the 17th century. For a long time confusion about their zoological pedigree ran riot and they were even believed to have connections with certain protozoa now known as gregarines. Nowadays, many helminthologists prefer to give them the status of a phylum (table 1.1). The general morphology of mature acanthocephalans is shown in figs. 1.37–1.46. The retractile proboscis, after which the worms are named, is the most characteristic organ. In nearly all species, the proboscis is armed with hooks (figs. 1.37, 1.40)

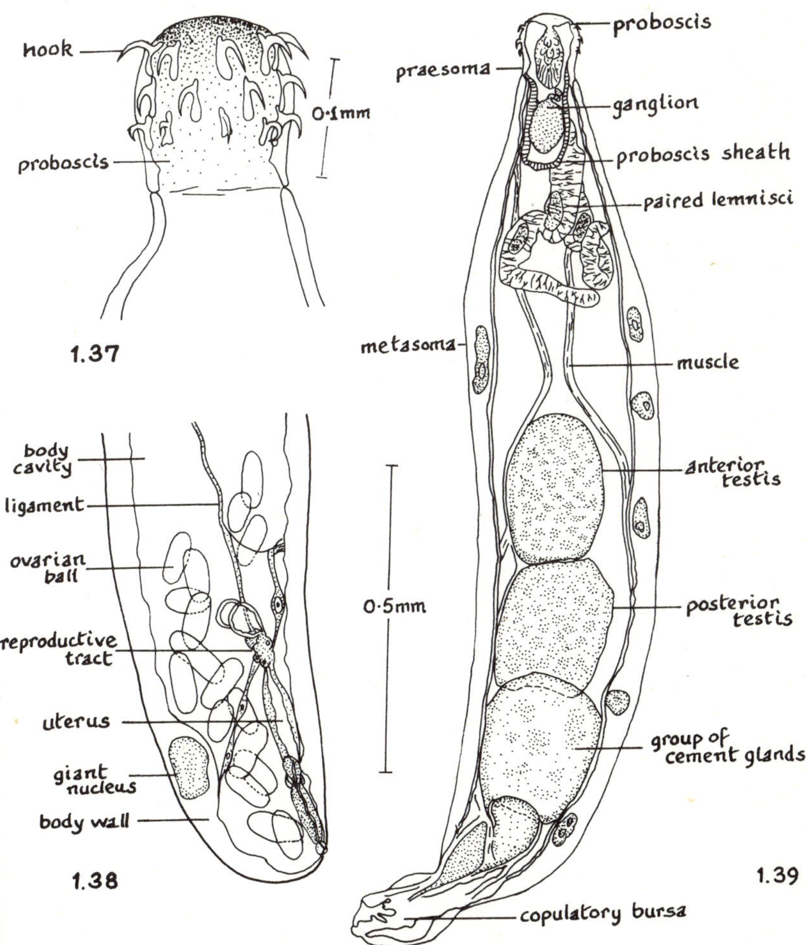


Figs. 1.37–1.39. *Ostospiniferoides chandleri* (Acanthocephala) (after Bullock, 1969, *J. Parasit.*, **52**, 735). 1.37. Proboscis. 1.38. Posterior end of a female worm. 1.39. Male.

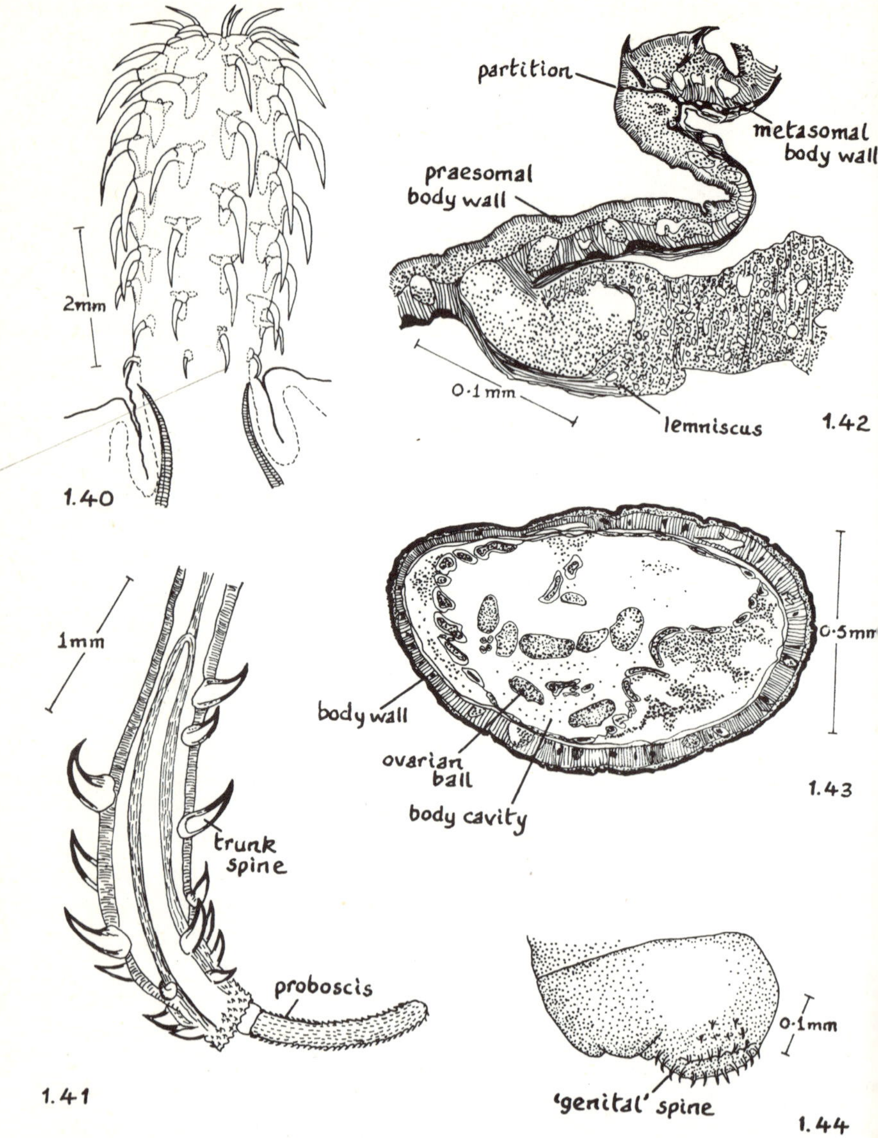


Figs. 1.40–1.44. Features of the morphology of mature acanthocephalans. 1.40. Proboscis of *Acanthocephalus anguillae* (after Luhe, 1911). 1.41. The large trunk spines of *Rhadinorhynchus horridus* (after Hyman, 1951, *The Invertebrata*, III). 1.42. Section through the junction of the praesomal and metasomal body wall of *Polymorphus minutus* (after Crompton, 1963, *Parasitology*, **53**, 663). 1.43. Transverse section through the body of an unmated female *P. minutus* (after Crompton, 1963, *Parasitology*, **53**, 663). 1.44. Trunk spines ('genital') at the posterior end of *Corynosoma* sp. (after Hyman, 1951, *The Invertebrata*, III).

and, if the worms are placed in warm saline and examined under a microscope, the proboscis can be observed as it is withdrawn and extruded from the proboscis sheath. During one cycle of proboscis activity, the hooks change position, from being on the outside and facing backwards to being on the inside and facing forwards.

As far as we know, all acanthocephalans are endoparasites. They are dioecious worms which mature and mate in the alimentary tract of vertebrates. Many species are about 5–30 mm long, the female worms generally being longer than the males. Female *Macracanthorhynchus hirudinaceus* from domestic pigs may be about 650 mm long, and females of *Nephridacanthus longissimus* from the aardvark, measuring from about 830 to 1000 mm, are probably the longest acanthocephalans known. *Corynosoma hamanni* is a species in which the males are larger than the females. An acanthocephalan worm does not possess an alimentary tract and its body wall (figs. 1.45, 1.46), like that of tapeworms, is adapted for the uptake of nutrients. They also possess a body cavity, in which the reproductive organs are suspended. Several aspects of the morphology and functioning of their reproductive organs appear to be unique in the animal kingdom. The paired organs known as the lemnisci (figs. 1.39, 1.42) are also unique and diagnostic of members of the phylum.

Unlike flukes, tapeworms and roundworms, the spiny-headed worms have never presented a major health hazard to man and domestic animals. This state of peaceful coexistence may account for the fact that little intensive research has been carried out on their biology. Recent Russian publications on the treatment of acanthocephalan infections in ducks suggest that some problems are developing or are expected. Perhaps these parasites may hinder fish-farming projects or schemes for wildlife conservation and management.

## 1.3. *Nematoda—roundworms*

The nematodes are one of the most interesting and successful groups of animals. The cylindrical shape of many species and the uniform nature of their anatomy may give the impression that they are all rather similar. Nothing could be further from the truth. Free-living nematodes live in almost every aquatic and terrestrial microhabitat from the poles to the tropics. As many as $3 \times 10^9$ individuals have been estimated to live in the top 76 mm (3 inches) of an acre of temperate soil, and half that number in the top 20 mm of an acre of shore-line sand. Plant-parasitic species are equally abundant, and man's crops are devastated by the unseen legions of subterranean worms. Reliable calculations of the economic losses to crops are

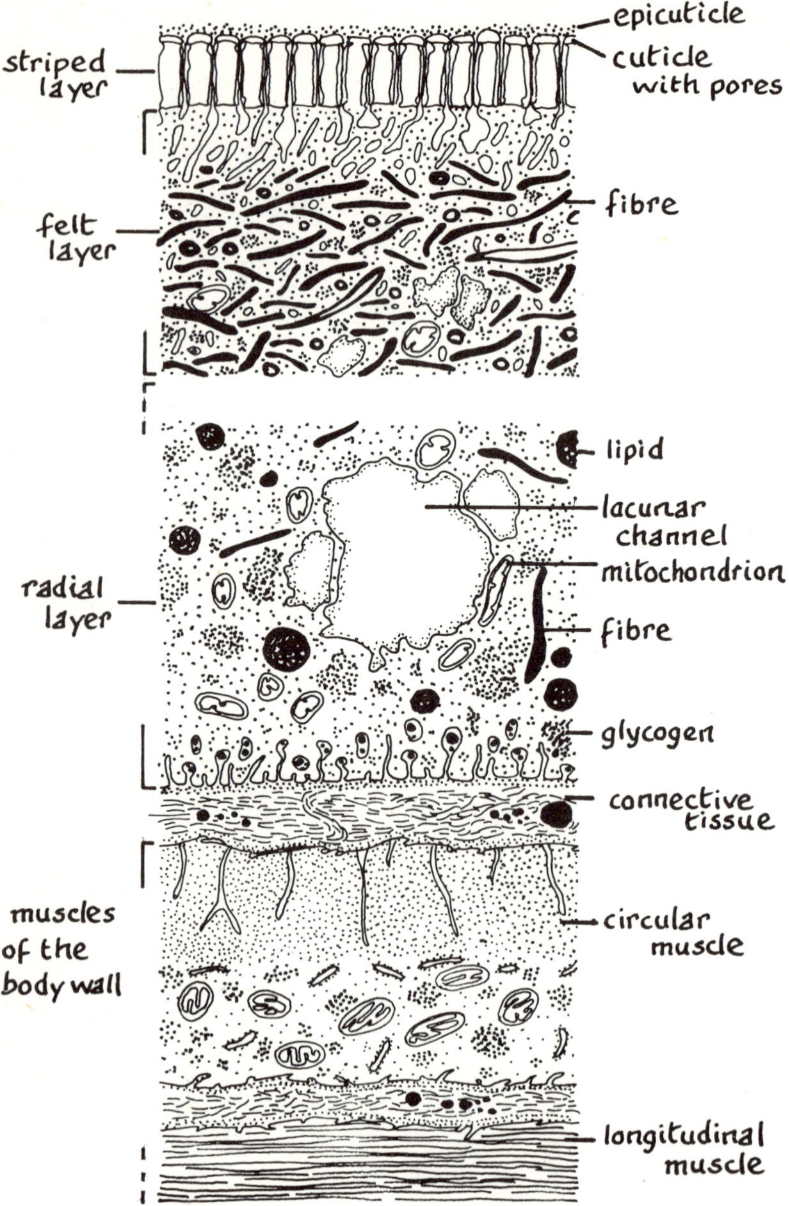


Fig. 1.45. Diagrammatic reconstruction, based on electron micrographs, of the metasomal body wall of an adult *Polymorphus minutus* (Acanthocephala) (after Crompton and Lee, 1965, *Parasitology*, **55**, 357).

difficult to make and accept, but plant-parasitic nematodes have been accredited with depriving farmers in the USA of 25% of their harvest. Many of the species which live in animal hosts are equally injurious, and one could argue that animal-parasitic nematodes have caused mankind almost as many problems as the mosquitoes, tsetse flies and their relatives. The distribution and abundance of nematodes on the earth testifies to their ecological and physiological diversity.

Some biologists consider that the earth is inhabited by at least 500 000 species of nematode. About 10 000 species have been studied and named to date, and many of these live in animals. Most species of

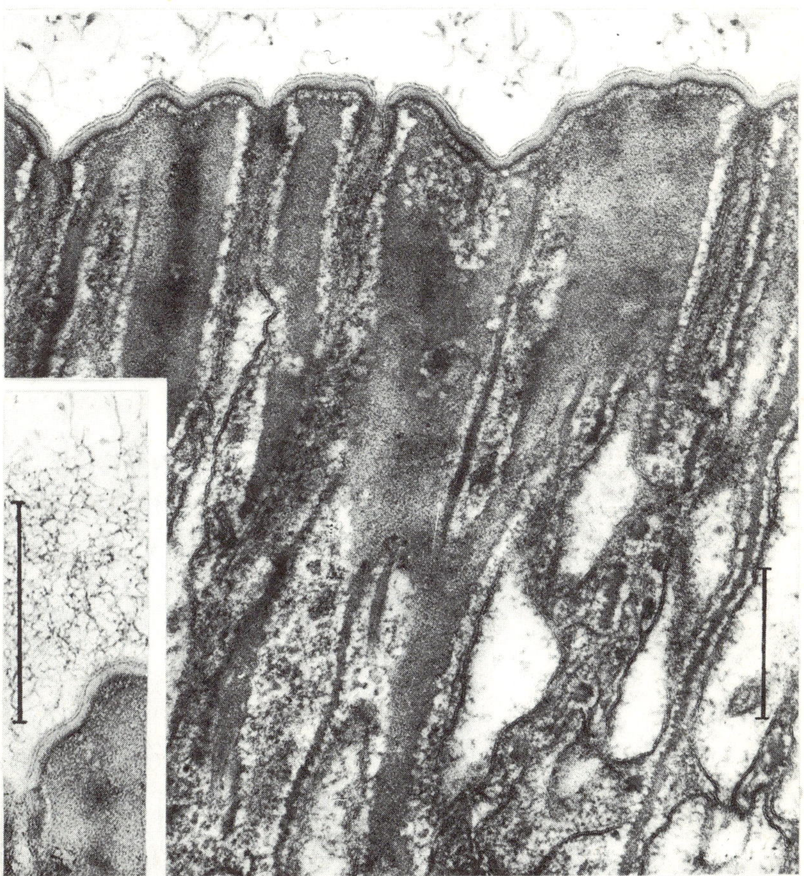

Fig. 1.46. Transmission electron micrographs of the surface layers of the metasomal body wall of an adult *Moniliformis dubius* (Acanthocephala). The scale represents approximately 0.5 $\mu$m. The inset shows a filamentous deposit which can sometimes be detected on the outer surface of the body wall.

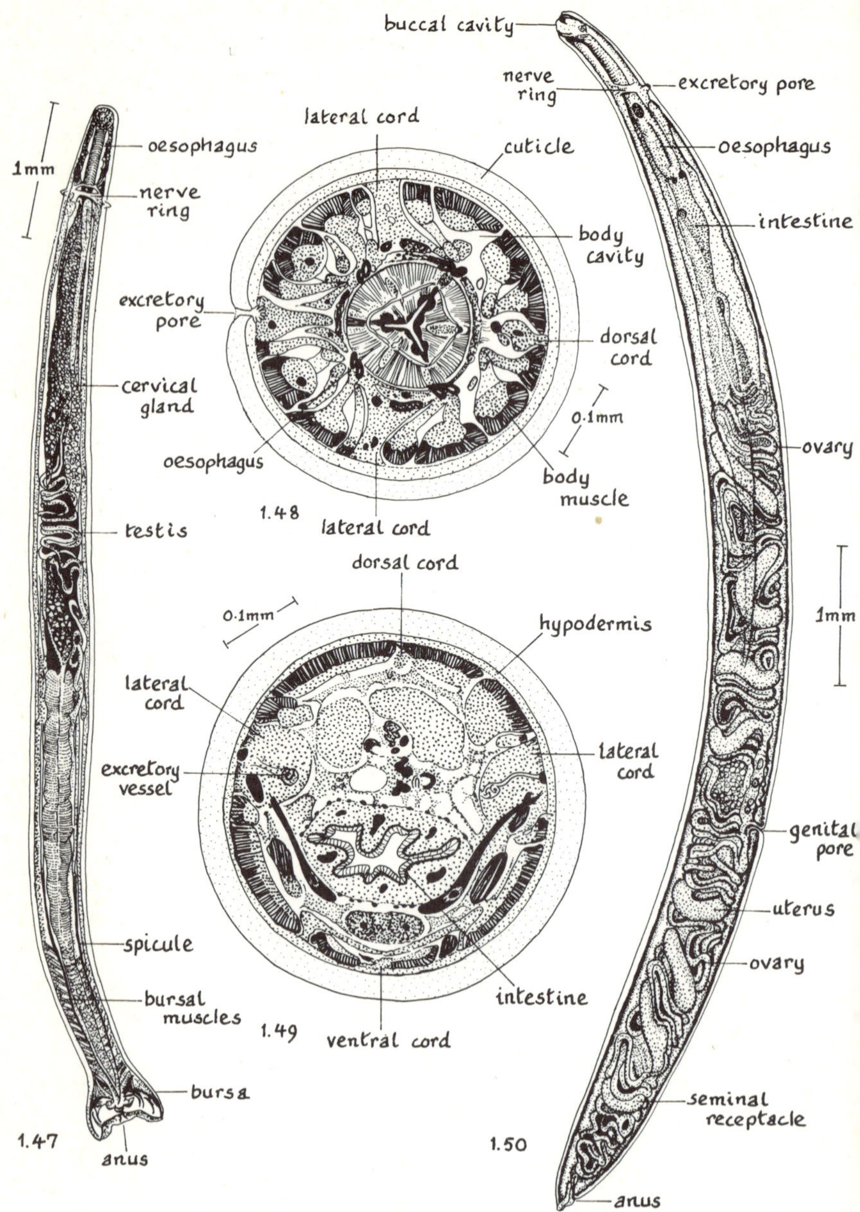


Figs. 1.47–1.50. Features of the morphology of adult nematodes illustrated by reference to the hookworm *Ancylostoma duodenale* (after Looss, 1905). 1.47. Adult male. 1.48. Transverse section through the region of the excretory pore. 1.49. Transverse section through posterior body of an adult male. 1.50. Adult female.

nematode are small, but the range of lengths is from about 200 $\mu$m to many centimetres. The longer nematodes are usually the animal-parasitic species. It is perhaps unfortunate that *Ascaris* has been adopted by so many educational courses to illustrate nematode biology. *Ascaris* is very convenient for study because of its world-wide distribution and large size, but its size and mode of life make it rather atypical of nematodes in general, in the same way that a whale is a somewhat atypical representative of the mammals.

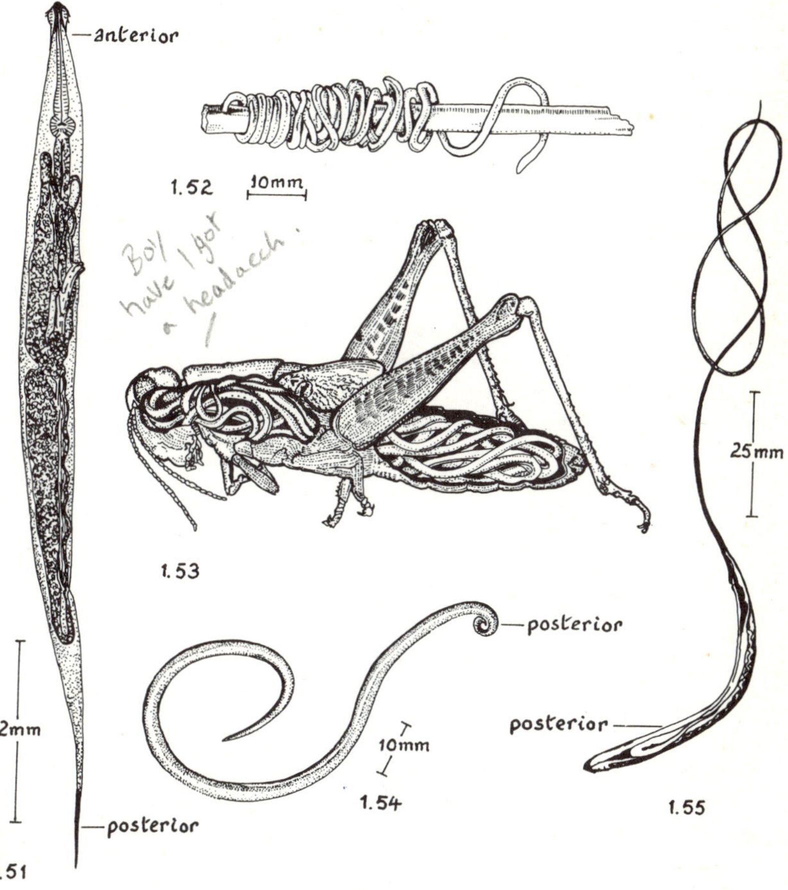


Figs. 1.51–1.55. Various nematodes. 1.51. Adult female *Enterobius vermicularis* (after Hyman, 1951, *The Invertebrata*, III). 1.52. Adult *Dracunculus medinensis* trapped and wound on a match stick (after Cholodkowsky, 1899). 1.53. Grasshopper infected with an immature *Agamermis decaudata* (after Hyman, 1951, *The Invertebrata*, III). 1.54. Adult male *Ascaris lumbricoides* (after Cholodkowsky, 1899). 1.55. Adult female *Trichuris* sp. (after Hyman, 1951, *The Invertebrata*, III).

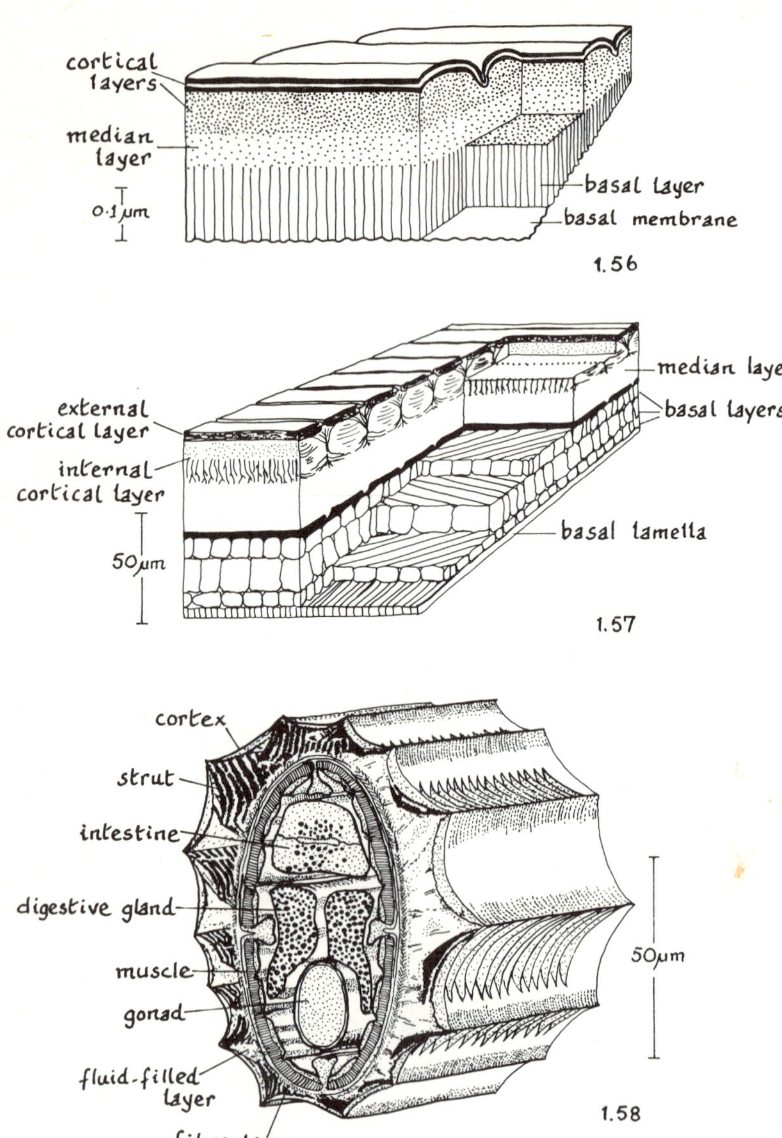


Figs. 1.56–1.58. Features of the cuticle and structure of nematodes. 1.56. Diagram of the cuticle of a typical larva (after Bird, 1971, *The Structure of Nematodes*). 1.57. Diagram of the cuticle of adult *Ascaris lumbricoides* (after Bird, 1971, *The Structure of Nematodes*). 1.58. Stereogram of a thick section taken from the middle region of adult *Nippostrongylus brasiliensis* (after Lee, 1969, *Symp. Brit. Soc. Parasit.*, **7**, 3).

Morphological features of nematodes are illustrated in figs. 1.47–1.60 by reference to animal-parasitic species. Typical roundworms are spindle-shaped or thread like, unsegmented, bilaterally symmetrical animals with a body cavity. The cuticle (figs. 1.56–1.58) is produced by the hypodermal layer, which is prominent in cross section as four longitudinal hypodermal cords (figs. 1.48, 1.49). The cuticle is renewed during moulting, which normally occurs four times before the adult stage is reached. The muscles of the body wall lie longitudinally, and each muscle cell consists of a contractile and non-

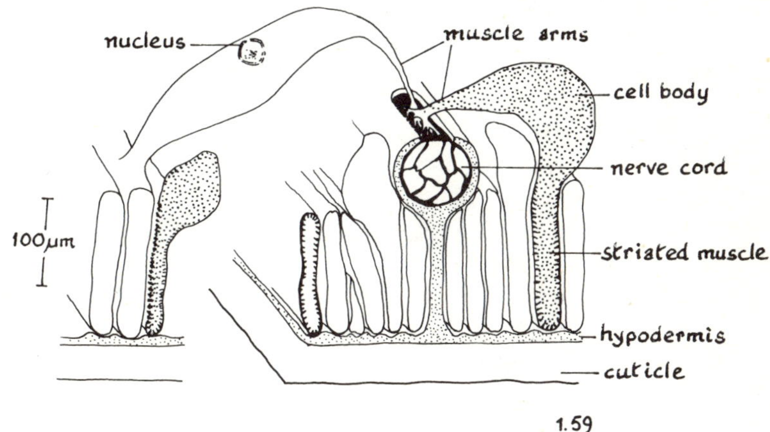


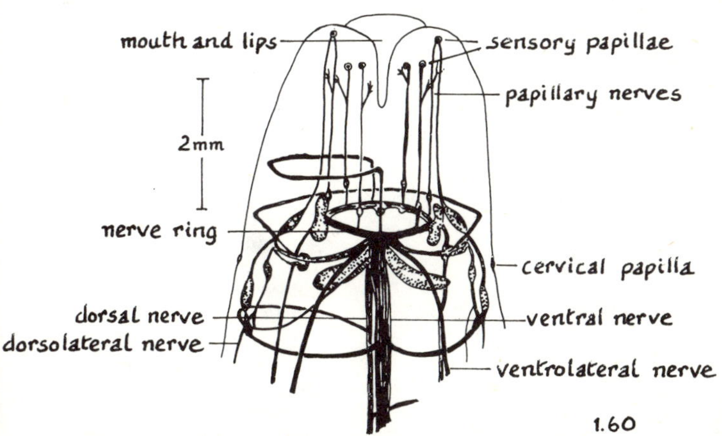


Figs. 1.59–1.60. Features of the nervous system of *Ascaris lumbricoides* (Nematoda). 1.59. Diagram showing the body muscle cells and their connexions with a nerve cord (after Bird, 1971, *The Structure of Nematodes*). 1.60. The anterior part of the nervous system (after Hyman, 1951, *The Invertebrata*, III).

contractile portion. The innervation of the muscles is achieved by a muscular connection making contact with the nerve rather than by a nerve axon running to the muscle (fig. 1.59). In addition, while the ultrastructure of the contractile elements is reminiscent of insect or vertebrate striated muscle, the results of electrophysiological studies of *Ascaris* muscle suggest that the muscles of the nematode body wall may function like the smooth muscle of the vertebrate small intestine.

A nematode may also be recognized by the nature of the muscular oesophagus or foregut with its triradiate lumen (fig. 1.48). The characteristic circumoesophageal ring of the nervous system is also associated with the anterior part of the alimentary tract. Nematodes are usually dioecious and the females are often larger than the males. In the females, the gonads have their own opening from the body to the exterior, but in the males they open into the rectum near the copulatory structures (fig. 1.47).

The main purpose of this chapter has been to describe some of the diagnostic features of different parasitic worms and to present some of the morphological interpretations which are now generally accepted by many parasitologists. Before we press on to read of observations made with the electron microscope and study results obtained by gas chromatography, liquid scintillation counting and other sophisticated techniques, we should pause to reflect. It is easy to ridicule those of our scientific forefathers who gave tapeworms anthropomorphic features†, and believed they arose by spontaneous generation‡ and argued, perhaps with tongue in cheek, that they disliked music§. Whatever their opinions, these early observers transmitted in their writings their fascination with what they saw. The plethora of information which now floods upon the senses of the modern parasitologist must not be allowed to quench his curiosity and drown his enthusiasm for the worms.

† Fig. 1.27, which was taken from a book published in 1721, is attributed to Malpighius.

‡ Aristotle (4th century BC), who achieved so much in establishing scientific method and knowledge, thought that tapeworms were inborn and arose from the putrefying intestinal contents of the foetus within the uterus of the mother. Ideas like these prevailed for centuries, even after Redi demonstrated in the 17th century that maggots could not be found in meat unless the parent flies laid eggs on the meat.

§ Goeze (18th century) observed that, in several cases of people known to be harbouring tapeworms, abdominal discomfort was felt in church when the organ began to play. He surmised that the pains stemmed from the agitation of the unhappy tapeworms. He also made many fine contributions to parasitology, including pioneer work on *Ascaris*.

# 2. Life cycles

In textbooks, the life cycles of parasitic worms are usually summarized by diagrams, which are as important to the parasitologist as are charts of metabolic pathways to the biochemist. The life-cycle diagram tells the parasitologist which hosts are involved; where the adult and developmental stages of the parasites are to be found; and how dispersal and transmission between hosts are likely to occur. Comparative studies of the life cycles of a group of parasites may aid in taxonomic studies and in the general problem of establishing phylogenetic relationships. It is not unreasonable to assume that parasites which infect similar hosts in a similar manner and sequence have had a similar evolutionary history. Information about the life cycle is most important when attempts are made to control those parasites which induce disease. Knowledge of the life cycle is the basis on which attempts are made to decide when a parasite will be most vulnerable to attack and when its host will be at least risk. This book is almost entirely about life cycles and our purpose here is to describe some of the concepts involved and to introduce some of the approaches to their study.

## 2.1. *Life cycles of helminths*

### 2.1.1. *Types of life cycle*

Self-explanatory information about the life cycles of monogeneans, digeneans, cestodes, acanthocephalans and nematodes is presented in figs. 2.1–2.5 respectively. Descriptions of the various developmental stages, which are mentioned by name in the figures, are presented in subsequent parts of this book and especially in Chapters 3 and 8.

As a rule, a parasite gives rise by reproduction to immature offspring which leave the original host. These offspring may be eggs or larvae, with or without surrounding envelopes. When the parasite eventually becomes established in the same type of host as the one from which it was discharged, without the obligatory involvement of any other host, the life cycle is said to be direct. Exceptionally, there are cases where the life cycle is direct but the adult stages are the ones entirely free from the host. Adults of the nematode *Agamermis decaudata* live in soil, where the eggs are laid by the females after copulation. Under the appropriate conditions, the eggs hatch and the larval stages wriggle up shoots of dew-soaked vegetation to which hungry grasshopper nymphs are attracted. The larval *Agamermis* then bores through one of the thinner regions of the cuticle of the feeding insect and grows at a phenomenal rate in the host's body cavity (fig. 1.53). After spending 1 to 3 months in the grasshopper, the nematode abandons its host and returns to the soil, where further development occurs before reproduction can take place. A similar life cycle is experienced by *Mermis nigrescens*, which is a close relative of *Agamermis* and is known in the British Isles as the thunderworm, because the adults can be seen climbing on stems and leaves after a summer thunderstorm. *Mermis* differs from *Agamermis* in that it appears to be capable of parthenogenetic reproduction and its eggs, as opposed to larvae, are swallowed by the insect hosts. However, in the majority of helminth life cycles that are direct, the parasite undergoes a phase of sexual reproduction within its single host. In all types of life cycle, the host which harbours the mature reproducing parasite is termed the definitive host.

Many parasites are unable to complete their development and re-enter their definitive hosts without a phase of larval development and sometimes multiplication in at least one type of intermediate host. Life cycles involving one or more intermediate hosts are said to be indirect. Digenean flukes are interesting in that all known species have a strict requirement for a gastropod mollusc as one intermediate host, while some require two or even three intermediate hosts. For example, *Alaria mustelae* is a small digenean which matures amongst the intestinal villi in mink in North America. The following phases of the life cycle occur in an aquatic snail, a frog and a small rodent. Laboratory studies indicated that if mink ate infected frogs, the fluke developed in the mink to the stage normally found in the small rodent and sexual maturity was not achieved. So the life cycle is normally completed in the wild only when mink eat infected small rodents.

Sometimes, particularly in cases in which the definitive host is a sizable predator, completion of the life cycle is aided by a transport or paratenic host (fig. 2.4). The participation of such a host appears not to involve an essential phase of larval development but rather to increase the chances of successful transmission. For example,

*Centrorhynchus aluconis* is an acanthocephalan which matures in the small intestine of birds of prey. Its eggs develop in terrestrial insects as far as the cystacanth, which is the stage infective to the definitive host. It is to be expected that predatory birds will become infected with *C. aluconis* on eating insects harbouring cystacanths. The chances, however, of infections of *C. aluconis* becoming established in such hosts will be increased if they also catch rodents which serve as paratenic hosts. After the rodent has eaten an infected insect, the cystacanth of *C. aluconis* is not digested, but becomes encysted in and among the mesenteries of its new host. No growth or development of the parasite occurs, but the definitive host becomes infected when it devours the rodent.

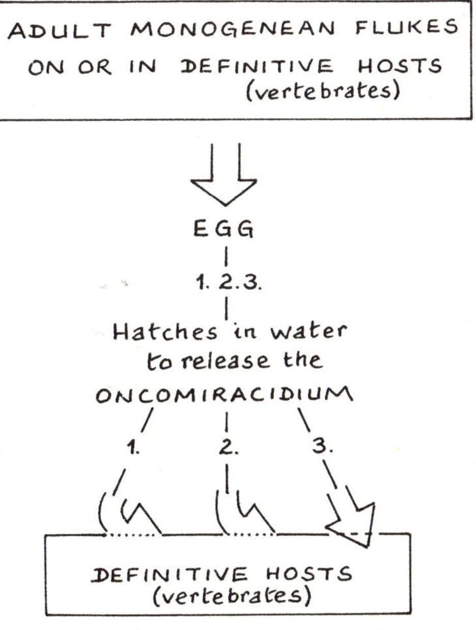


Fig. 2.1. Chart showing an outline of the life cycles of three species of monogenean fluke. 1. *Diclidophora merlangi*. 2. *Entobdella soleae*. 3. *Polystoma integerrimum* (development in synchrony with breeding cycle of host).

## 2.1.2. *Host specificity*

Diagrammatic representations of life cycles as shown in figs. 2.1–2.5 do not emphasize the host specificity of parasitic worms. The common pinworm, *Enterobius vermicularis*, appears to be restricted to man and to have no other host in which it can mature and reproduce. In

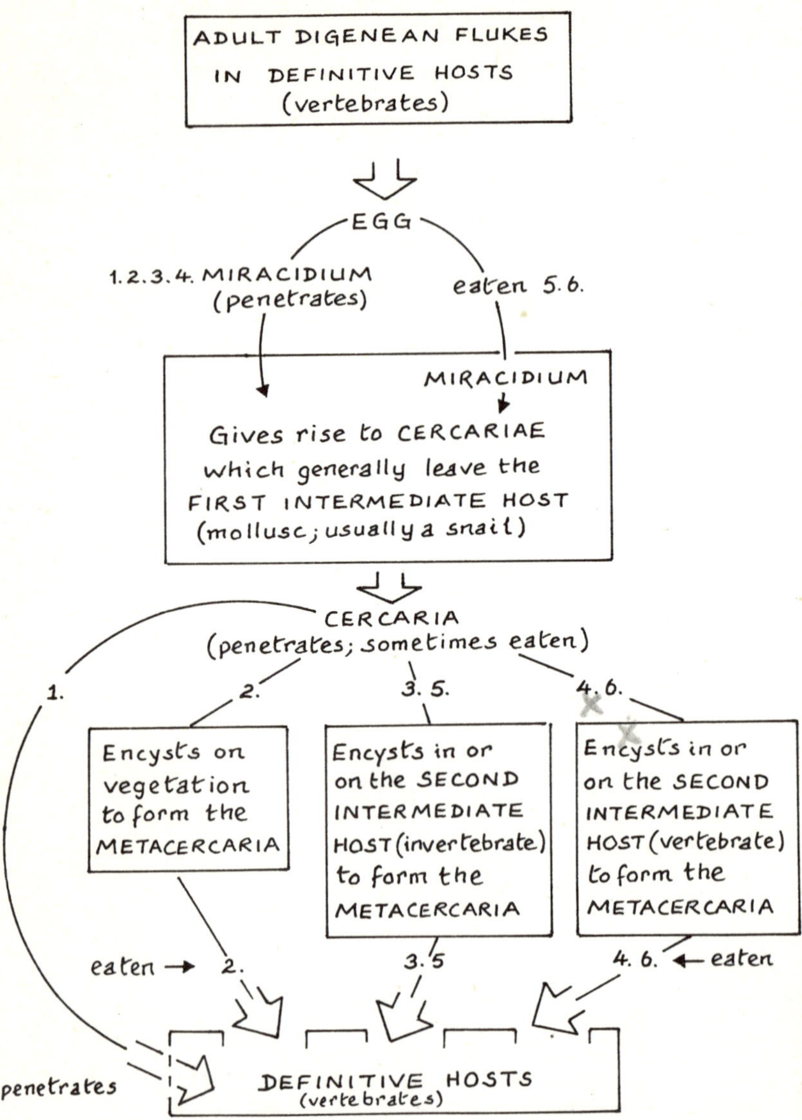


Fig. 2.2. Chart showing an outline of the life cycles of six species of digenean fluke. 1. *Schistosoma mansoni*. 2. *Fasciola hepatica*. 3. *Parorchis acanthus*. 4. *Diplostomum phoxini*. 5. *Haematoloechus medioplexus*. 6. *Cryptocotyle lingua*.

×D. phoxini is an unencysted metacercar

contrast, the oriental blood fluke, *Schistosoma japonicum*, may complete its life cycle in man, cattle, water-buffalo, horses, sheep, goats, cats, dogs, pigs, rodents and probably in other mammals. *Schistosoma japonicum* is a serious agent of disease in man, and its relatively low host specificity presents a problem for its eradication. Even if treatment is available for patients in an area where the parasite occurs, the threat of infection will always be present unless domestic animals are destroyed. In many rural areas, livestock represents a community's main economic asset, and its loss might cause greater hardship than the parasitic disease.

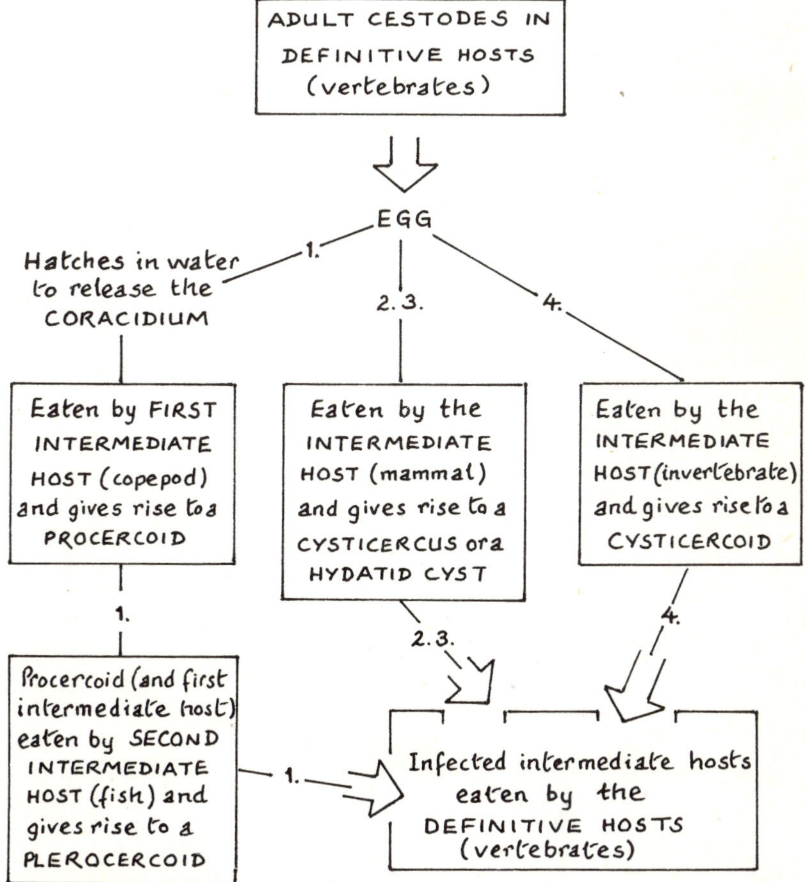


Fig. 2.3. Chart showing an outline of the life cycles of four species of cestode. 1. *Diphyllobothrium latum*. 2. *Taenia saginata* (cysticercus). 3. *Echinococcus granulosus* (hydatid cyst). 4. *Hymenolepis diminuta*.

Published lists of the hosts in which different helminths have been found may not always convey useful information about specificity because some hosts may support a certain amount of growth of a given parasite but not its reproduction. These hosts may represent a cul-de-sac for the parasite. *Polymorphus minutus* appears to have been found in the small intestine of over 80 species of bird, but it is not known whether it can reproduce and release viable eggs from all these hosts. This question cannot be solved until infections of known age are studied in the laboratory with birds of known pedigree and history as hosts. It is fundamental that taxonomic procedures and conclusions about the identification of helminths should be accurate

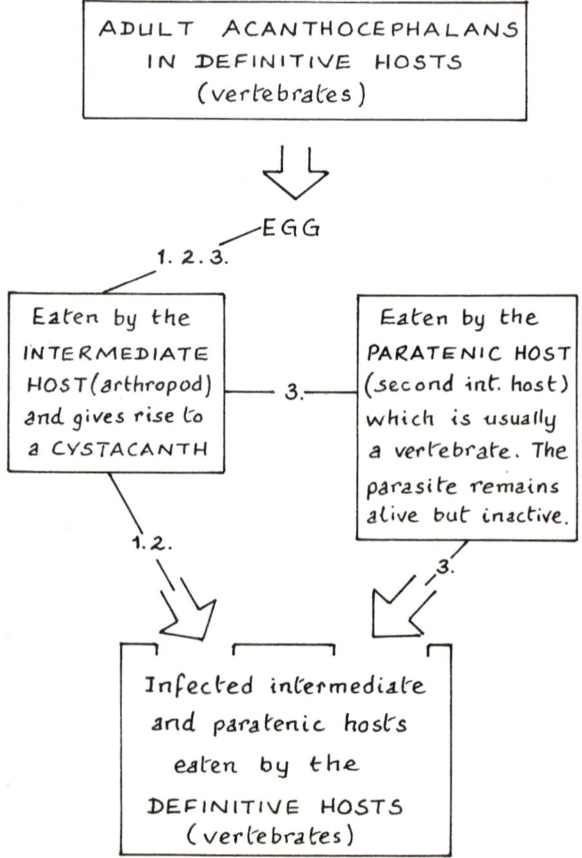


Fig. 2.4. Chart showing an outline of the life cycles of three species of acanthocephalan. 1. *Moniliformis dubius* (insect intermediate host). 2. *Polymorphus minutus* (crustacean intermediate host). 3. *Neoechinorhynchus cylindratus* (crustacean first intermediate host, fish second intermediate host).

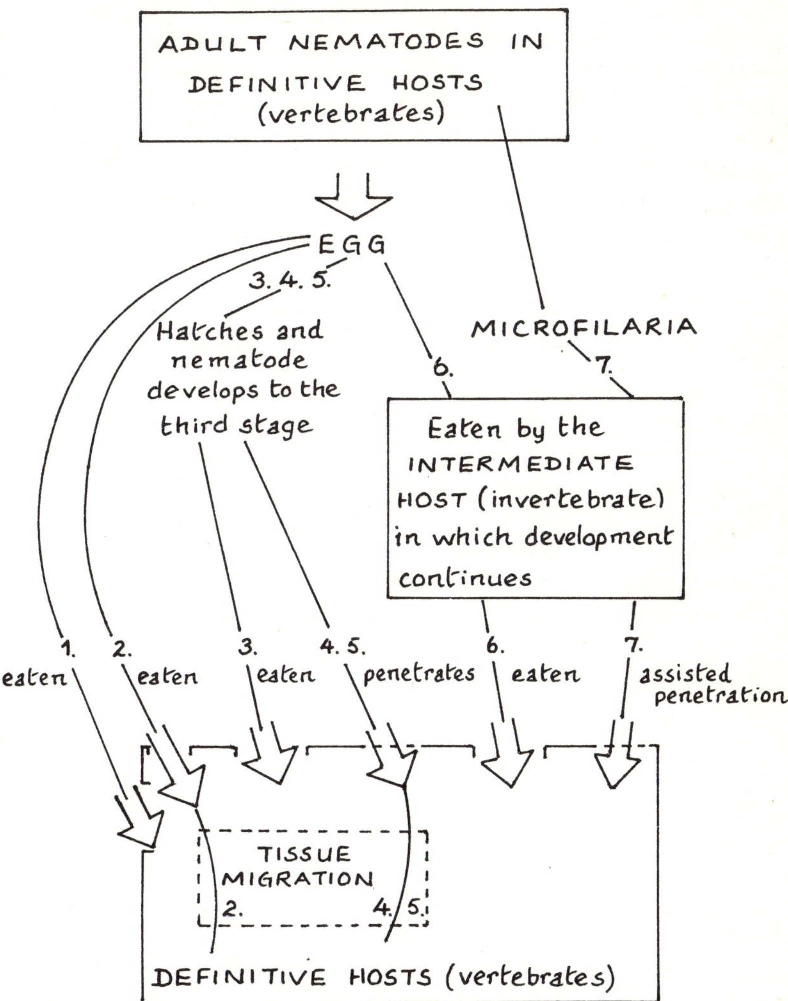


Fig. 2.5. Chart showing an outline of the life cycles of various species of nematode. 1. *Enterobius vermicularis*. 2. *Ascaris lumbricoides*. 3. *Haemonchus contortus*. 4. *Nippostrongylus brasiliensis*. 5. Hookworms (*Ancylostoma* and *Necator*). 6. *Gongylonema neoplasticum*. 7. *Wuchereria bancrofti*.

if host specificity is to be understood. Before identification, many helminths have to be treated with histological fixatives and other chemicals. The choice of a fixative is critical and placing worms from the same population in different fixatives often results in varying degrees of shrinkage of the cells and tissues. Thus, an artificial difference in parasite size may be introduced into a homogeneous population. The taxonomist must be as conscientious about his methods as any experimental scientist.

The matter of the host specificity of helminths has been complicated further by the recognition of strains and races of both hosts and parasites. Morphological differences between strains may not be significant, but other differences, which probably reflect physiological variation, are known. For example, there are several groups of species of planorbid (ram's horn) snail belonging to the genus *Bulinus* which are actual or potential intermediate hosts for the blood fluke *Schistosoma haematobium* in Africa. Snails from the *B. truncatus* group are generally found north of the equator while snails from the *B. africanus* group are usually found to the south. Curiously, the specificity of *S. haematobium* for hosts of one group or the other is so strong that some workers have proposed that the parasite should be considered as two species. *Schistosoma haematobium* is suggested as the name for the strains dependent on the *B. truncatus* group of snails and *S. capense* for those dependent on the *B. africanus* group. Clearly the existence of strains of a parasite and of varying degrees of host specificity does nothing to simplify the work of the aetiologist and epidemiologist.

The innate and acquired resistance of hosts to parasites is obviously a major factor which contributes to specificity, but so are other facets of host–parasite relationships. Many of these features will emerge in later chapters and a few examples here may help to alert the mind. Tapeworms of the order Tetraphyllidea (table 1.1) show a high degree of specificity for the species of elasmobranch fish in which they mature. The morphology of the mucosa of these fish is characteristic for each species, and when the morphology of the scolices of the tapeworms is examined it appears that each scolex has become modified to interlock with a particular mucosal surface. In some tapeworms, the scolex is fully developed by the time the parasite enters its definitive host. *Echinococcus granulosus* becomes established in the small intestine of suitable carnivores after the ingestion and exposure of the infective stage to digestive secretions including bile. The results of studies *in vitro* suggest that the detergent action of the bile salts may provide some activating stimulus for the parasite.

Herbivores, in contrast, are generally unsuitable hosts for *E. granulosus* and it is known that the bile from rabbits or sheep dissolves the surface of this tapeworm. Finally, the distribution and behaviour of hosts should not be ignored in considerations of host specificity. For example, laboratory work has established that *Schistosoma mansoni* will develop in white mice, but in nature these rodents are not found in the water where the cercariae are swimming.

## 2.2. *Ecological approaches to the study of life cycles and parasitism*

### 2.2.1. *Environmental relationships within the host*

Ecology may be regarded as the study of the relationship between an organism and its environment, where the environment is defined according to its physical and biotic factors, or in terms of the weather, food, other organisms present and places in which to live. This arbitrary and convenient concept can be applied to endoparasites whose environment is a living host. For example, the environment of a mature acanthocephalan is to be found in the morphology of the alimentary tract of its host, in the physicochemical conditions prevailing during and between phases of digestion, and in the activities of the microbes and other parasites. The requirements of mature blood flukes are supplied by the composition and properties of the circulating venous blood of susceptible hosts. A fuller understanding of the complexity of parasitism has probably emerged from attempts to combine knowledge of a parasite's physiology with information about the conditions existing in its living environment. This approach also emphasizes the variety of environments which a parasite experiences during its life cycle. For example, the tapeworm *Diphyllobothrium latum* develops first in the body cavity of a crustacean and then among the muscles of a fish, before reproduction occurs in the small intestine of a mammal (fig. 2.3).

### 2.2.2. *Environmental relationships between hosts*

Parasitologists must also consider how the life cycle of a parasite is integrated into the ecological relationships of its hosts. The distribution, abundance, food preferences, migrations and other features of the host, including its position in food webs, are factors which probably influence the dispersal and transmission of a parasite and, therefore, the perpetuation of the species. Recently, mathematical techniques have been used to study populations of parasites during their life cycles. An example of the approach is shown in outline in fig. 2.6 which describes the life cycle of *Transversotrema patialense* in

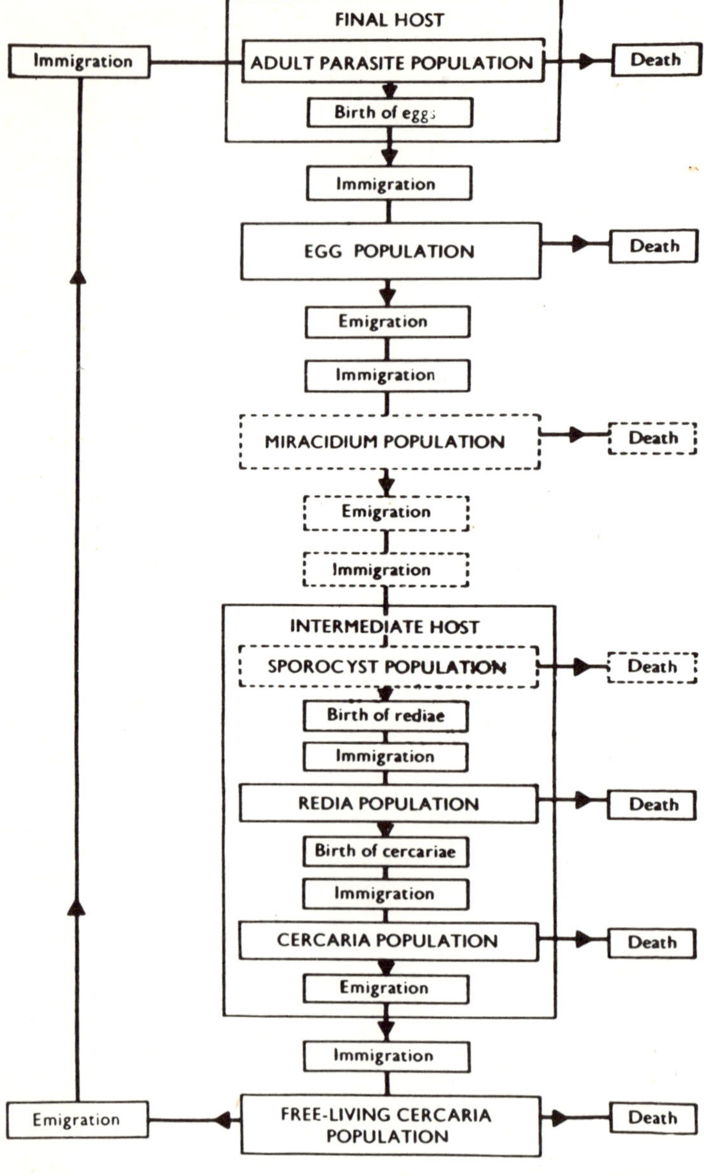


Fig. 2.6. Diagrammatic flow chart of the population processes involved in the life cycle of a transversotrematid fluke (Digenea). The boxes delineated by dotted lines indicate that these parasitic larval stages and population processes have not as yet been conclusively demonstrated (from Anderson and Whitfield, 1975, *Parasitology*, **70**, 295).

terms of population dynamics. This digenean fluke is unusual in that the adults are ectoparasitic on fish, which becomes infected when attacked by cercariae (fig. 3.29). The life cycle is ideal, however, for population studies because the adult worms can be counted and observed directly on their hosts without the observer having to make too great an intrusion into their environment. Many investigations of parasitism are difficult because the relationship between the parasite and the host is in a state of equilibrium which is inevitably disturbed by experimental intervention.

## 2.3. *The course of infection*

The duration of the association between a population of helminths and their host is called the course of the infection, which may be divided into the prepatent and the patent periods†. The prepatent period extends from the beginning of the infection until the release of reproductive stages begins. The patent period is the time during which these stages are being liberated. The numbers of infective stages, the susceptibility and resistance of the host and the size and developmental state of populations of parasites within the host are some of the factors which influence the course of an infection, in addition to other environmental features within and without the host. The flow chart for *T. patialense* (fig. 2.6) postulates how recruitment and loss occur within the population at different stages of the life cycle, and provides a framework for analysis.

The methods of cybernetics, or systems analysis, may also be employed to investigate how a host–parasite relationship proceeds

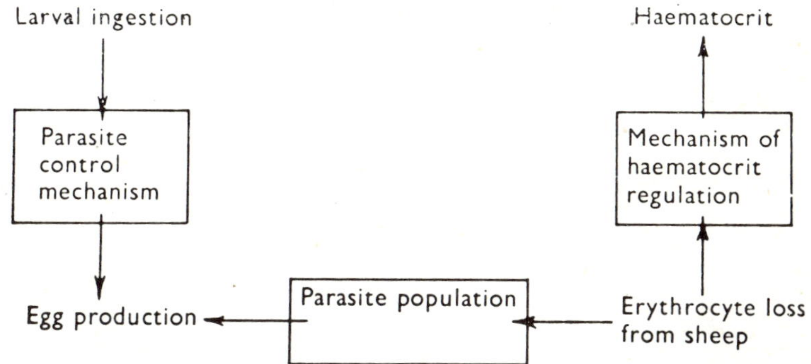


Fig. 2.7. The three principal components (black boxes) of the sheep–*Haemonchus contortus* (Nematoda) interaction (from Ratcliffe, Taylor, Whitlock and Lynn, 1969, *Parasitology*, **59**, 649).

† 'Patent' means lying open to view.

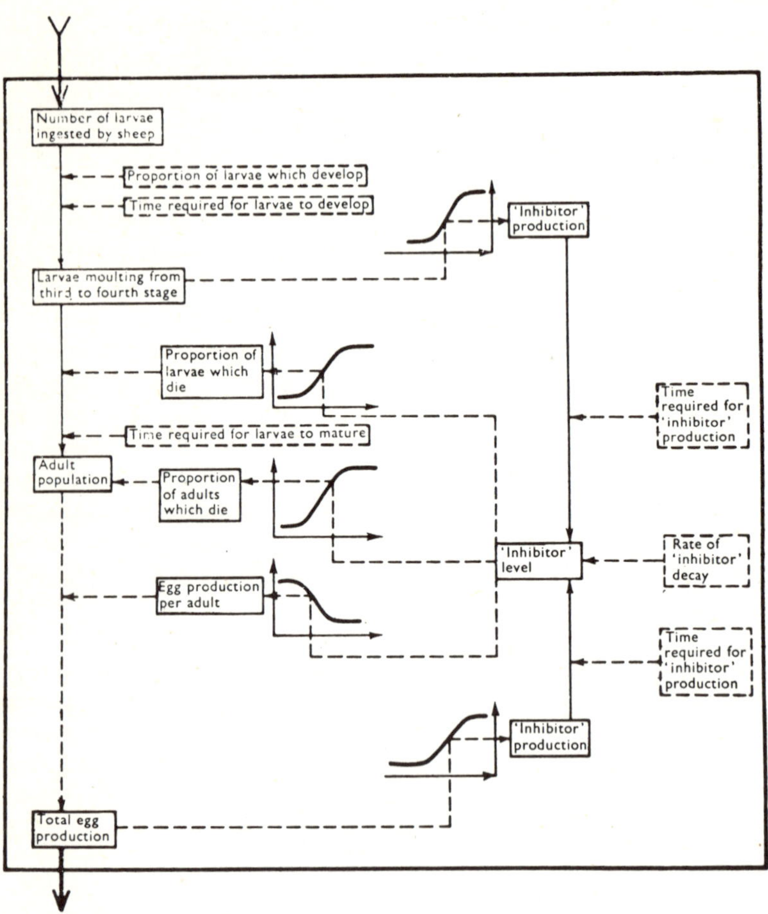


Fig. 2.8. A postulated model of the parasite control mechanism which may operate during infections of *H. contortus* (Nematoda) in sheep (fig. 2.7). The continuous lines represent flows of information. Variables which have to be specified in the input data of the computer programme of the model are enclosed in dashed boxes. The symbol showing a graph denotes where provision has been made for some sort of function relating two variables (from Ratcliffe, Taylor, Whitlock and Lynn, 1969, *Parasitology*, **59**, 649).

during the course of an infection. This approach has been developed at Cornell University in New York during studies of the nematode *Haemonchus contortus* (fig. 2.5), which infects and damages sheep. The adult parasites live in the sheep's abomasum where the female worms produce many eggs which eventually reach the pasture. Larvae hatch from the eggs and moult twice before becoming infective to sheep. On being ingested by the host, the larvae undergo two more moults, the worms attain maturity, and the cycle is completed as eggs are discharged. Under optimum conditions the entire cycle can occur in 20 days, but in winter in New York the cycle is arrested because the eggs and larvae cannot survive in the fields. When the host–parasite relationship is flourishing, however, the blood-sucking activities of the worms initiate haemorrhage from the abomasal wall and the sheep become anaemic and weak.

Many observations have been made on flocks of sheep which have been experimentally infected with *H. contortus*. These findings and the development of the disease cannot be understood until valid hypotheses have been formulated and tested. Cybernetics makes use of a conceptual device known as the black box which represents the unknown factors operating during the transformation of inputs into outputs. The three principal components, or black boxes, of the relationship between *Haemonchus* and sheep are shown in fig. 2.7. Detailed information about larval ingestion, which represents an input, and egg production, which represents an output, can be obtained, and models of the type depicted in fig. 2.8 can be postulated to explain what may be happening within the host. Similar models can be constructed for the other black boxes, and a mathematical representation of the host–parasite relationship and the development of the disease can be obtained. Experiments can then be designed to see if the mathematical predictions are realized.

# 3. Transmission and infection

The mechanisms which have evolved because they facilitate the transmission of parasitic helminths between hosts and ensure the establishment of infective stages on or in their hosts are as ingenious and intricate as any of the activities of living organisms. Most attempts to generalize about the varied modes of transmission and infection will fail to please everyone. Nevertheless, some form of classification and some definitions are necessary for purposes of communication.

The term 'transmission' will be used to encompass the events occurring from the departure of an organism from one host until contact is made with the next host in the cycle. 'Infection' will be considered to be the means by which the parasite becomes established and physiologically committed to dependence on the next host. It should not be forgotten that the role of the host in transmission and infection is often as important as that of the parasite.

Transmission and infection are usually discussed together since both involve the infective stages of the parasite. Transmission may occur as a result of four general processes. These are: (a) contamination, (b) the behaviour of infective stages, (c) the involvement and behaviour of intermediate hosts and to a lesser extent (d) the behaviour of adult helminths. Some of these processes apply to the transmission and infection of ectoparasitic worms.

The infection of hosts by most species of endoparasite usually occurs by either the oral or the cutaneous route, although some infective stages may be drawn into gills and lungs, or may even cross the mammalian placenta from the mother to the foetus. All aspects of transmission and infection, however, depend on the natural ecological interplay of hosts, potential hosts, and infective stages in time and place. In the following discussion, the adaptations of a selection of host–parasite relationships are described to illustrate certain features of transmission and infection.

## 3.1. *Morphology of infective stages*

Aspects of the morphology of a variety of infective stages of parasitic

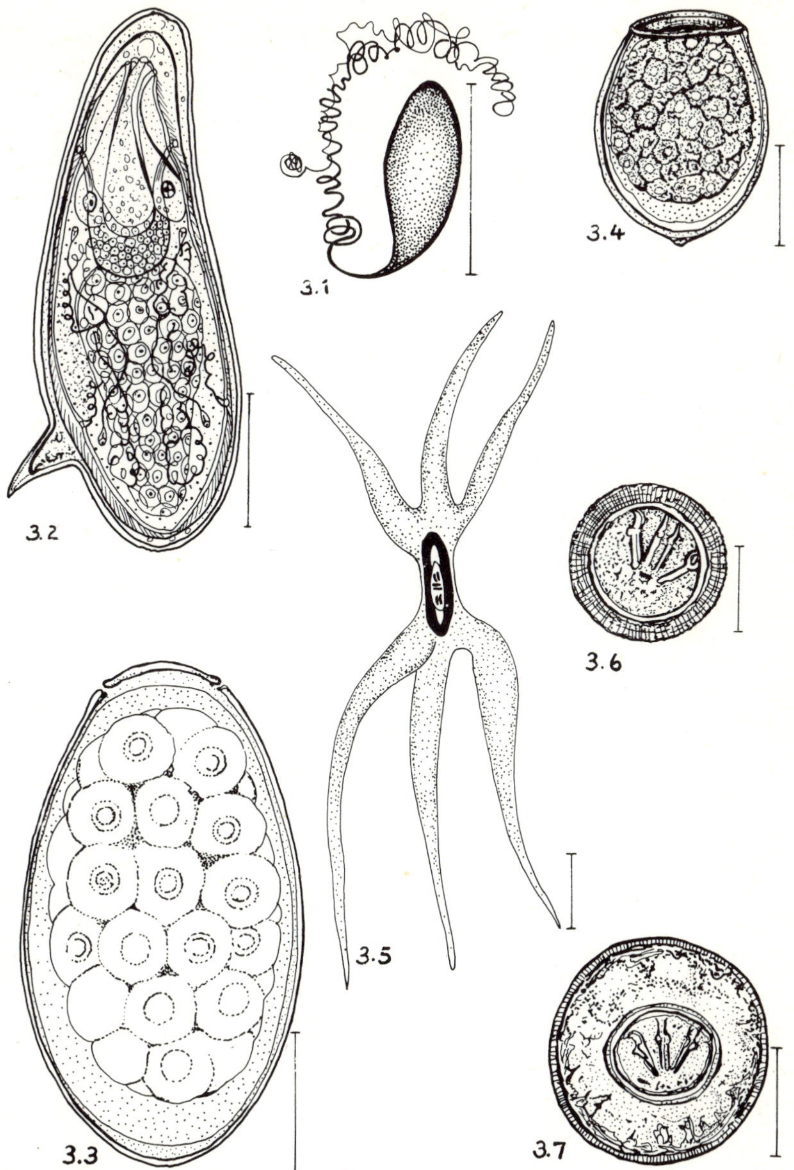


Figs. 3.1–3.7. Eggs of platyhelminths. The scale for each figure represents about 25 μm. 3.1. Monogenea. *Diplozoon paradoxum* (after Zeller, 1872). 3.2 and 3.3. Digenea. 3.2. *Schistosoma mansoni*. 3.3. *Fasciola hepatica*. 3.4–3.7. Cestoda. 3.4. *Diphyllobothrium latum*. 3.5. *Diorchis* sp. (after Jarecka, 1961, *Acta Parasit. Pol.*, **9**, 409). 3.6. *Taenia saginata*. 3.7. *Hymenolepis diminuta*. The purpose of these figures and of figs. 3.8–3.16 is to show something of the variety of form and size of helminth eggs.

worms are presented in figs. 3.1–3.43. The stages shown in these figures include examples from direct life cycles and from indirect cycles involving two, three and four hosts. In some cases, for example *Hymenolepis* spp., both the intermediate and definitive hosts are infected by stages which are ingested (figs. 3.7, 3.32). In other cases, for example *Schistosoma* (figs 3.18, 3.27), both hosts are infected by stages which penetrate the body surface, while in other cases, for example *Fasciola*, the intermediate host becomes infected through its skin, while the definitive host becomes infected through its alimentary tract (fig. 3.36).

## 3.2. *Transmission*

### 3.2.1. *Contamination*

Contaminative transmission is mainly achieved by the casual acquisition of the infective stage by the host. The developmental cycles of most parasites that are transmitted by this method involve the production of large numbers of infective stages which are resistant to adverse environmental conditions. It will be demonstrated however, that the production of many resistant infective stages is often a feature of other forms of transmission.

Estimates of the numbers of infective stages produced by parasitic worms are given in table 3.1. Most of these figures have been obtained under experimental conditions and may not be accurate for worms living in a natural situation. For example, the egg production of a female *Moniliformis* of about 5 000 eggs (fig. 3.8) per day (table 3.1) lasts for about 15 weeks. This information was estimated from primary infections of not more than 12 worms in male rats which were free from other species of parasite and which were receiving unlimited quantities of water and a highly nutritious diet. Furthermore, the rats were housed under constant conditions without interference from other rats, predators or competitors. The egg production of *Moniliformis* may be very different when the worms form a part of a fluctuating population in wild rats which are also hosts to other parasites and which are experiencing normal environmental stresses. In fact, the results of other investigations, discussed elsewhere in this book, will show how the fecundity and patent period of a worm may be affected by the size of the population, by other parasites and by the nature of the host's diet.

In addition to the production of many infective eggs and the larval stages arising directly from them (figs. 3.17–3.25), the developmental cycles of digenean flukes and some species of cestode include the

TABLE 3.1. *Estimations of the reproductive output of some endoparasitic worms. (See table 8.1 for information about life expectancy of worms.)*

| Parasitic worm | Egg production (per worm per day) | |
|---|---|---|
| DIGENEA | | |
| *Schistosoma mansoni*[a] | 100 | (hamster) |
| CESTODA | | |
| *Echinococcus granulosus*[b] | 600 | (dog) |
| *Hymenolepis diminuta* | 200 000 | (rat) |
| *Taenia saginata* | 720 000 | (man) |
| ACANTHOCEPHALA | | |
| *Moniliformis dubius* | 5 000 | (rat) |
| NEMATODA | | |
| *Ascaris lumbricoides* | 200 000 | (pig) |
| *Enterobius vermicularis* | 11 000 | (man) |
| *Wuchereria bancrofti* | 12 500 MF[c] | (man) |

[a] Each egg may give rise asexually to 100 000 cercariae.
[b] Each egg may give rise to a hydatid cyst in which polyembryonic development produces millions of scolices in a cyst the size of an orange.
[c] MF are microfilariae (figs. 3.23–3.25).

asexual production of cercariae (figs. 3.26–3.30) and scolices (fig. 3.35) by polyembryony (table 3.1). Thus it appears that organisms with a high reproductive capacity have been selected during the evolution of parasitism. The production of so many infective stages may seem prodigal and inefficient, but it ensures the survival of the parasites. Some idea of the losses of infective stages may be obtained by realizing that if each of the 200 000 eggs produced each day by a single *Hymenolepis* during a period of 18 months (table 3.1) gave rise to a mature tapeworm, about 120 tons of tapeworm tissue would be synthesized. Similarly, if each cercaria developing by polyembryony from a single egg of *Schistosoma* (table 3.1) gave rise to an adult worm, about 60 tons of blood fluke tissue would be generated.

Another factor which appears to assist transmission is the resistance of many infective stages to physical and chemical conditions in the environment. These conditions may be encountered in the host's environment or in different organs and tissues of the host which are unsuitable for the growth of the parasite. Some of the structural adaptations of resistant infective stages are indicated in figs 3.1–3.16.

The resistant properties of the eggs of *Ascaris* (fig. 3.11) are remarkable and probably contribute to the enormous biological

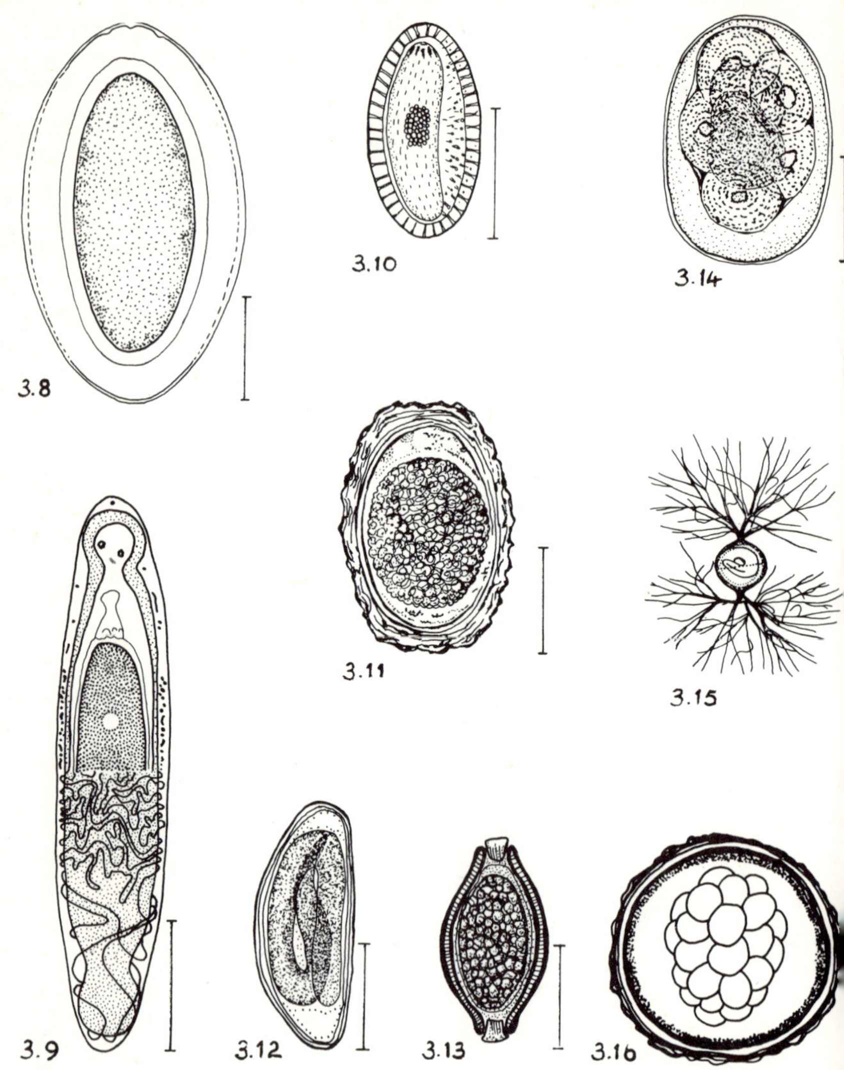


Figs. 3.8–3.16. Eggs of Acanthocephala and nematodes. The scale for each figure represents about 25 $\mu$m. 3.8–3.10. Acanthocephala. 3.8. *Moniliformis dubius* (after Whitfield, 1971, *Parasitology*, **62**, 35). 3.9. *Polymorphus minutus* (after Whitfield, 1973, *Parasitology*, **66**, 387). 3.10. *Paulisentis fractus* (after Cable and Dill, 1967, *J. Parasit.*, **53**, 810). 3.11–3.16. Nematoda. 3.11. *Ascaris lumbricoides*. 3.12. *Enterobius vermicularis*. 3.13. *Trichuris trichiura*. 3.14. Hookworm (*Ancylostoma* and *Necator*). 3.15. *Mermis subnigrescens* (after Christie, 1929, *J. exp. Zool.*, **53**, 59). 3.16. *Toxocara canis* (after Christenson, 1950, In: *Introduction to Nematology*). Note the complexity of the eggshells and the possible adaptations of the eggs. The egg of *Diplozoon* (3.1) may become entangled in waterweed and that of *Mermis* (3.15) appears to have a 'byssus' for attachment to vegetation.

success of this nematode. When the eggs of *Ascaris* are released from the female worm, they contain a zygote which begins to cleave so that the morula, blastula and gastrula stages, followed by the first and second larval stages, occur in the host's environment and often in association with sewage. Under optimal conditions in temperate regions, this embryonic and post-embryonic development takes about 20 days and involves one ecdysis. It has been reported that these processes can occur even when the eggs are immersed in 0.3% carbolic acid, 9% sulphuric acid, 14% hydrochloric acid, 8% glacial acetic acid, 12% formalin, normal sodium hydroxide or saturated solutions of mercuric chloride, copper sulphate and copper acetate. Cytoplasmic cleavage has been observed to continue under pressures of up to 800 atmospheres, and development continued after centrifugation at 400 000 *g* for one hour. The ability of the parasite to survive such reagents and forces in addition to the stresses of the natural environment, sometimes for several years, is probably directly related to the properties of the egg shell. Fortunately, the infectivity of the eggs is destroyed by relatively short periods of exposure to sunlight. There has been some controversy about the number of layers in the egg shell of *Ascaris*, but at least three layers are undoubtedly present. The inner layer is referred to as the lipid or ascaroside layer. It is about 0.6 μm thick and is composed of about 75% lipid and 25% protein. An inner lipid layer is a common component of the egg shells of many species of nematode. The middle layer of the egg of *Ascaris* is about 1 μm thick and is a mixture of chitin and protein. In biological materials, the function of chitin appears to be analogous to that of steel rods in reinforced concrete or of the filamentous meshwork in fibreglass structures. The outer or vitelline layer is probably composed mainly of protein. With the electron microscope, the outer surface of the vitelline layer appears to be bounded by a plasma membrane. A gelatinous, acid-mucopolysaccharide layer of variable thickness is often present on the eggs of *Ascaris* detected in faecal samples. This coating (fig. 3.11) is secreted by the wall of the worm's uterus. The other layers of the egg shell appear to originate from the enclosed embryonic tissue. The middle, chitin-containing layer is synthesized in response to the stimulus of fertilization. Not all eggs and encysted forms of helminths (figs. 3.1–3.16) are as hardy and resilient as the eggs of *Ascaris*.

### 3.2.2. *Behaviour of infective stages*

A general conclusion from observations made on the structure and biology of oncomiracidia (fig. 3.17), miracidia (figs. 3.18–3.20),

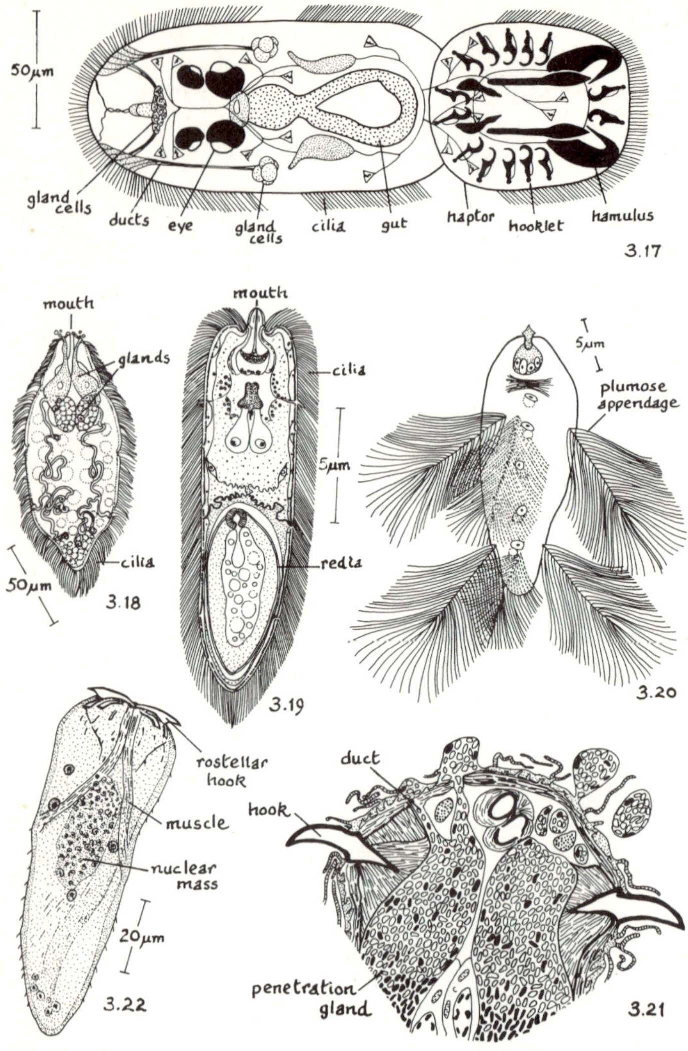


Figs. 3.17–3.22. Features of the morphology of some infective stages of parasitic worms. 3.17. Monogenea. Oncomiracidium of *Entobdella soleae* (after Kearn, 1971, In: *Ecology and Physiology of Parisites*). 3.18–3.20. Digenean miracidia. 3.18. *Schistosoma mansoni* (after Belding, 1958, *Basic Clinical Parasitology*). 3.19. *Parorchis acanthus* (after Rees, 1940, *Parasitology*, **32**, 372). 3.20. *Leucochloridomorpha constantiae* (after Baer, 1952, *Ecology of Animal Parasites*). Note that not all miracidia are ciliated and plumose; the miracidium of *Halipegus amherstensis* lacks cilia and possesses spines. 3.21. Cestoda. A diagram, based on electron micrographs, of part of the oncosphere (hexacanth) of *Hymenolepis diminuta* (after Lethbridge and Gijsbers, 1974, *Parasitology*, **68**, 303). 3.22. Acanthocephala. Acanthor of *Mediorhynchus grandis* (after Moore, 1962, *J. Parasit.*, **48**, 76).

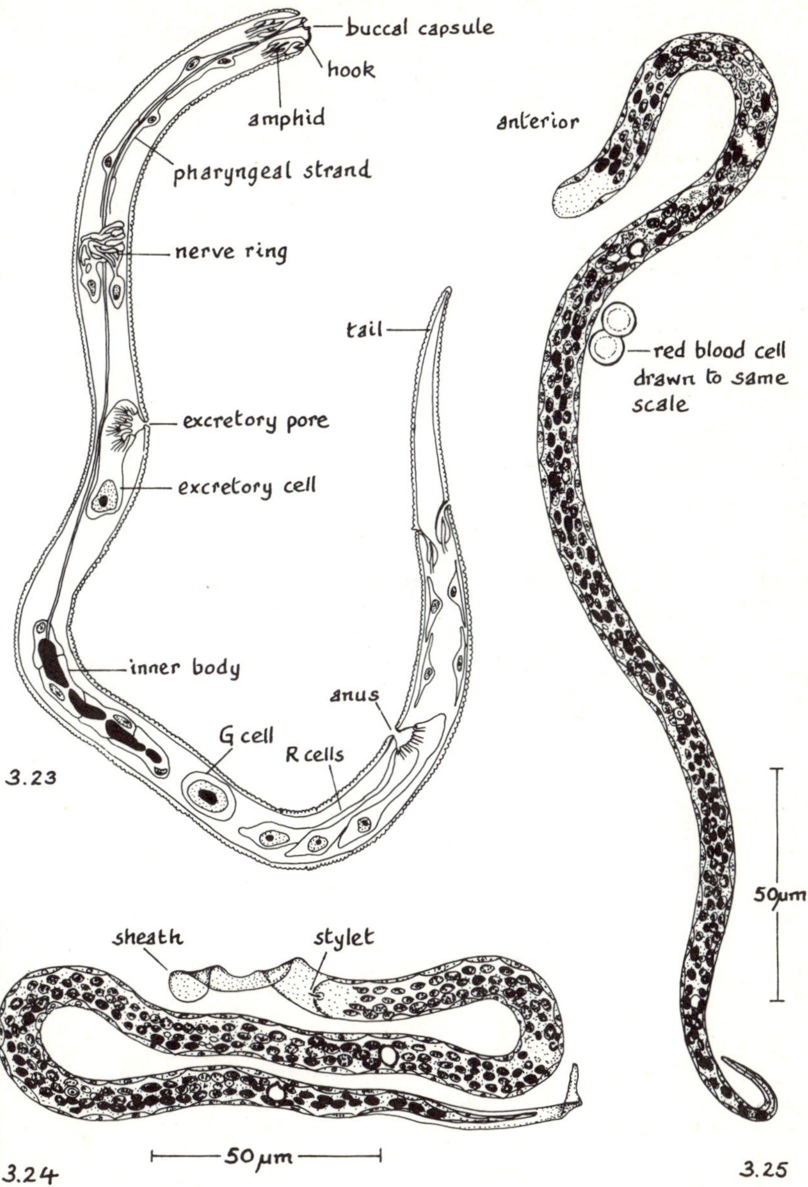


Figs. 3.23–3.25. Nematode microfilariae. 3.23. Basic microfilarial structure (after McLaren, 1972, Parasitology, **65**, 317). 3.24. *Wuchereria bancrofti* (sheathed). 3.25. *Onchocerca volvulus* (unsheathed).

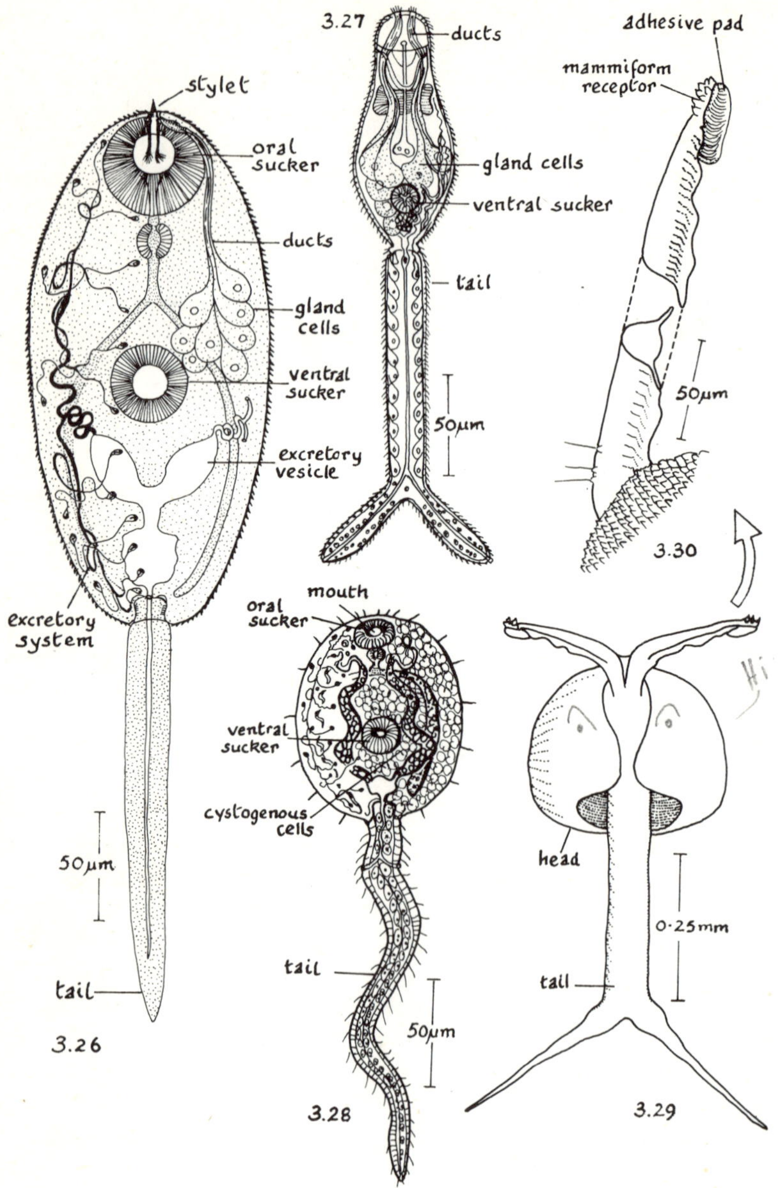


Figs. 3.26–3.30. Features of the morphology of some digenean cercariae. 3.26. *Plagiorchis megalorchis* (after Rees, 1952, *Parasitology*, **42**, 92). 3.27. *Schistosoma* spp. (after Belding, 1958, *Basic Clinical Parasitology*). 3.28. *Fasciola hepatica*. 3.29. *Transversotrema patialense* (after Whitfield *et al.*, 1975, *Parasitology*, **70**, 314). 3.30. Arm process of *T. patialense* (after Whitfield *et al.*, 1975, *Parasitology*, **70**, 314).

cercariae (figs. 3.26–3.30) and nematode larvae (figs. 3.23–3.25 and 3.41–3.43) is that certain aspects of their behaviour patterns contribute to transmission. Some of these stages appear to detect or seek out their hosts while others move into locations in the host's environment where contact is more likely to be made.

The oncomiracidia of monogeneans and the miracidia and cercariae of most digeneans appear to find their hosts after a brief period of active swimming. Some of these larval stages appear to prefer a particular depth of water or rate of water flow for their swimming and all the species so far studied appear to be unable to maintain themselves for more than 24 hours. Although our knowledge of the behaviour of parasitic flatworms is rather elementary, it appears that the behavioural responses of a given oncomiracidium, miracidium or cercaria result in its swimming in the zone of the habitat that is most likely to be occupied by a suitable host. This conclusion implies that as the host changes its distribution in its environment in response to various environmental factors or their combined effects, so will the behavioural responses of the parasites result in compensatory changes.

An example of the type of behaviour pattern which may ensure completion of transmission is that observed during an experimental study of the miracidia of *Schistosoma* (fig. 3.18). After these larvae have reached the environment of the gastropod host, *Biomphalaria glabrata*, they swim at a speed of about 120 mm $min^{-1}$ in smooth, straight lines. This scanning phase rapidly changes if the miracidium passes close to a suitable snail. The miracidia now perform a frantic underwater devil-dance, which probably represents a response to substances present in the snails or in the water in which they have been living. Critical tests using agar blocks impregnated with single chemicals have indicated that the miracidia of *S. mansoni* are much excited by butyric, glutamic and valeric acids amongst others. The change from scanning to the devil-dance is likely to increase the miracidium's chances of making contact with the snail. The efficiency of this form of host-finding in nature is unknown, but turbulence and currents will tend to disperse the stimulatory chemicals, and other ecological factors may affect the sensitivity of the parasites. It is known, however, that chemosensory reception is also important for the host-finding activities of other aquatic infective stages. The oncomiracidia of *Entobdella soleae* (fig. 3.17) are affected by substances associated with the skin epidermis of the fish host, the cercariae of *S. mansoni* and *S. haematobium* (fig. 3.27) respond to the free fatty acid fraction extracted from human skin and the cercariae of *Austrobilharzia terrigalensis* are stimulated by cholesterol obtained from the skin of avian hosts.

The infective stages of certain species of nematode, which have an obligatory free-living phase in the surface layers of the soil, often display behaviour patterns which are likely to enhance the opportunities for contact with the host. Some trichostrongylid nematodes, for example *Haemonchus contortus* (table 4.1), develop in the alimentary tract of herbivorous mammals which have acquired the parasites by swallowing herbage contaminated with infective third-stage larvae (fig. 3.42). In the period prior to attaining infective properties, the larval stages of the nematodes usually feed voraciously on soil micro-organisms but, on reaching the third larval stage, they stop feeding and climb to the tips of grass shoots, some of which are likely to be eaten by grazing sheep. The third-stage larvae of *Dictyocaulus viviparus* sometimes climb on to the sporangia of the fungus *Pilobolus kleini*, and are dispersed over the pasture when the sporangia explode. The infective, skin-penetrating, third-stage larvae of hookworms (fig. 3.41) and related nematodes also have a tendency to crawl to the highest points in their environment after an obligatory free-living phase in the surface layers of the soil.

The microfilarial larvae (figs. 3.23–3.25) of several species of nematode exhibit a marked rhythm with regard to their presence in the circulating blood of their definitive hosts. For example, the microfilariae of most strains of *Wuchereria bancrofti* are present in the blood of man only at night (fig. 3.44), while those of *Loa loa* are present only during the day (fig. 3.44). In monkeys, however, the periodicity of *L. loa* is reversed and most microfilariae are observed to be present in the blood at night. *Dirofilaria immitis* from dogs has a less pronounced rhythm in that some microfilariae are present in the blood by day but not as many as by night. Microfilariae are usually carried from host to host by biting flies in which they undergo an obligatory phase of development. The degree of synchronization between the presence of microfilariae in the circulating blood and the feeding activities of the insect hosts can be interpreted as a remarkable adaptation not only for transmission between definitive hosts but also for the infection of the intermediate hosts. The nocturnal periodicity of *W. bancrofti* has been known for many years, but only recently has it been discovered that the parasites accumulate in the lungs by day. Until this finding, an attempt was made to explain periodicity as a rhythmical effect of breeding. It was postulated that microfilariae were released every 24 hours from the adult female worms. Most of the offspring were assumed to die or be destroyed by the host's immune responses so that a cyclical parasitaemia would result. This idea collapsed when the numbers of circulating microfilariae were found to increase at a rate which could not be reconciled with either the fecundity of the worms or the powers of the host's defences. Furthermore, the microfilariae were found to be long lived. The general consensus now held to explain periodicity is that it stems from the behaviour of the parasites themselves; there are many delicate rhythmical changes in the physiology of the host to which the microfilariae might be sensitive, including deep-body temperature and vascular oxygen tension.

### 3.2.3. *Role of intermediate hosts*

Intermediate hosts participate in a variety of ways in the transmission of parasites. The behaviour of biting flies seeking a blood meal is an important factor in the transmission of filarial nematodes and it has been estimated that a person living in the Cameroons might expect about 14 000 bites a year from *Simulium damnosum*, the vector of *Onchocerca volvulus*. Some intermediate hosts, for example, flour beetles of the genus *Tribolium* which may contain cestode cysticercoids (fig. 3.32), inhabit stored cereals which are eaten by rats. Other intermediate hosts and paratenic hosts may form a part of the diet or be the main prey of the definitive hosts of the helminth in question. Insectivorous birds and mammals ingest a considerable range of invertebrates which may be potential intermediate hosts for helminths. In North America, belted kingfishers often harbour the digenean *Uvulifer ambloplitis*. Not surprisingly, the infection is acquired when the birds ingest metacercariae (see fig. 3.37) associated with the skin of rock bass, perch and sunfish.

The presence or activities of parasites may weaken intermediate hosts and render them more susceptible to capture by predatory definitive hosts. Perhaps the presence of relatively enormous burdens of larval tapeworms (*Ligula intestinalis*), which cause gross abdominal distension in roach (*Rutilus rutilus*), so impairs the swimming of the infected fish that they are more easily caught by the definitive hosts than are the uninfected fish. The metacercariae of digeneans of the genus *Diplostomum* frequently develop in the eyes and brains of freshwater fish, and it is possible that the infected hosts provide easy meals for piscivorous birds. The metacercariae of *Dicrocoelium dendriticum*, which is an economically important parasite of sheep, develop in the tissues of ants and may become encysted in the brain. Behavioural changes may be observed in infected ants, which begin to clamber up to the tips of grass shoots; presumably the probability

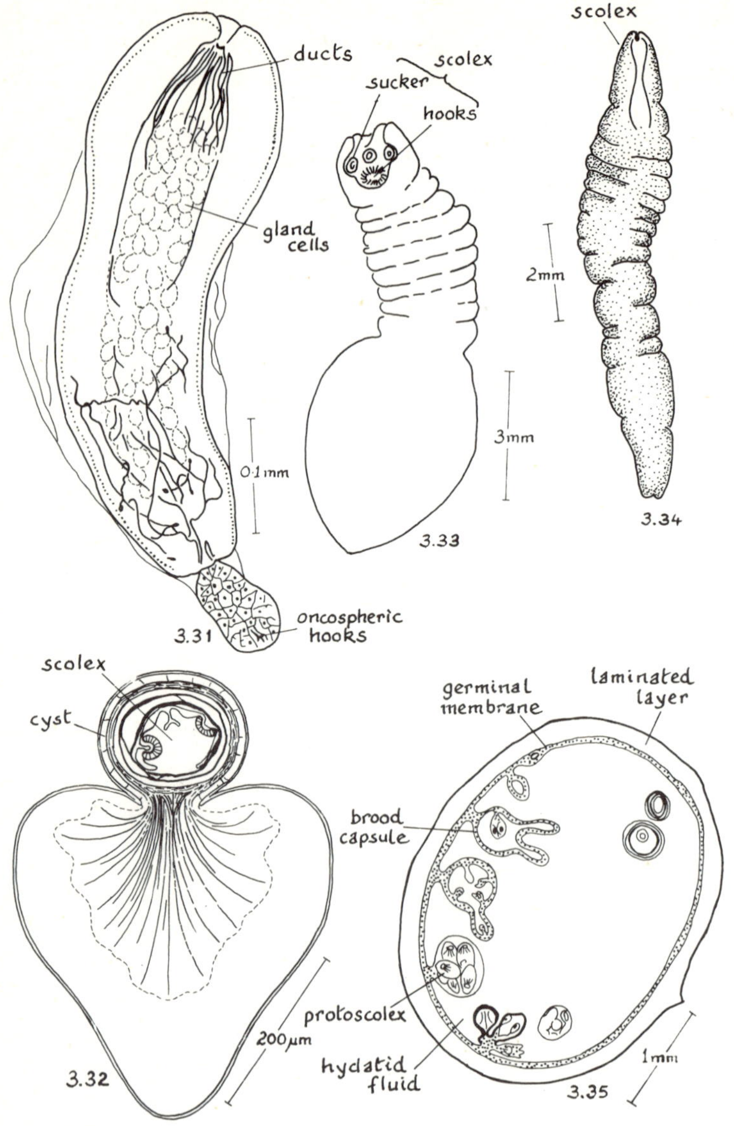


Figs. 3.31–3.35. Cestode larvae. 3.31. Procercoid of *Diphyllobothrium latum* (after Wardle and McLeod, 1952, *The Zoology of Tapeworms*). 3.32. Cysticercoid of *Hymenolepis microstoma* (after Caley, 1974, *Parasitology*, **68**, 207). 3.33. Cysticercus of *Taenia* sp. (after Freeman and Bracegirdle, 1971, *An Atlas of Invertebrate Structure*). 3.34. Plerocercoid of *Diphyllobothrium latum* (after Hyman, 1951, *The Invertebrata*, II). 3.35. Hydatid cyst of *Echinococcus granulosus* (after Wardle and McLeod, 1952, *The Zoology of Tapeworms*).

of sheep becoming infected is increased in consequence. *Dicrocoelium* is interesting in other respects because a terrestrial snail forms the first intermediate host and the cercarial stages do not swim to find the ants but reach them in balls of slime secreted by the snails.

In the cases cited above, investigations will probably show that increased contact between definitive and intermediate hosts arises from the gross pathological damage in the intermediate host caused by the parasite. Recently, extremely interesting changes have been detected in the behaviour of the amphipod *Gammarus lacustris* infected with the acanthocephalan *Polymorphus paradoxus*, which matures in the small intestine of dabbling ducks living on the shallow lakes of the aspen parkland in Alberta, Canada. Field observations indicated that infected *Gammarus* were often to be seen clinging to weed and flotsam at the water surface. The behaviour of infected and

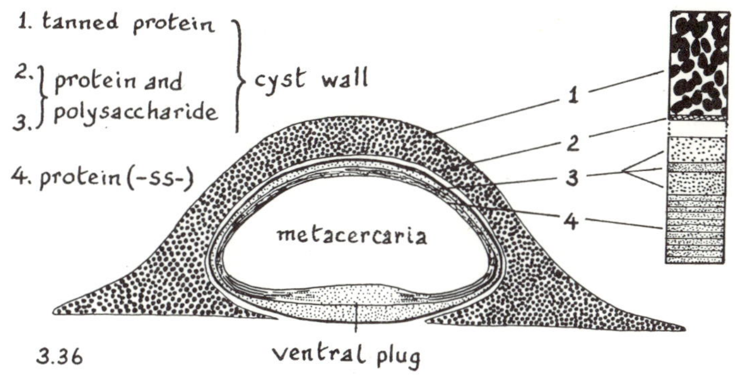


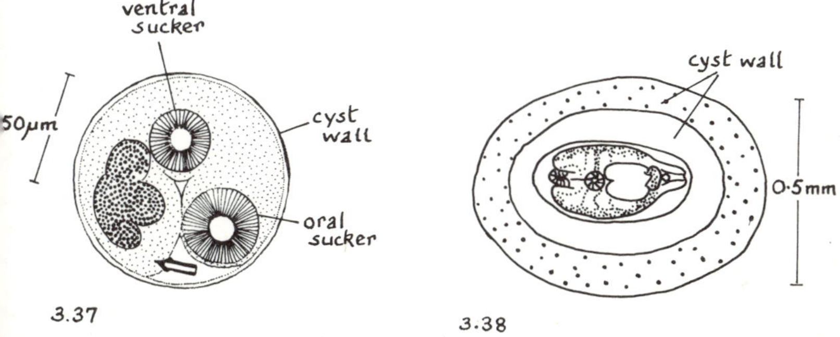


Figs. 3.36–3.38. Digenean metacercariae. 3.36. Multi-layered structure of the cyst wall surrounding the metacercaria of *Fasciola hepatica* (after Dixon, 1965, *Parasitology*, **55**, 215). 3.37. Metacercaria of *Plagiorchis megalorchis* (after Rees, 1952, *Parasitology*, **42**, 92). 3.38. Tetracotyle (form of metacercaria) of *Strigea elegans* (after Pearson, 1959, *J. Parasit.*, **45**, 155).

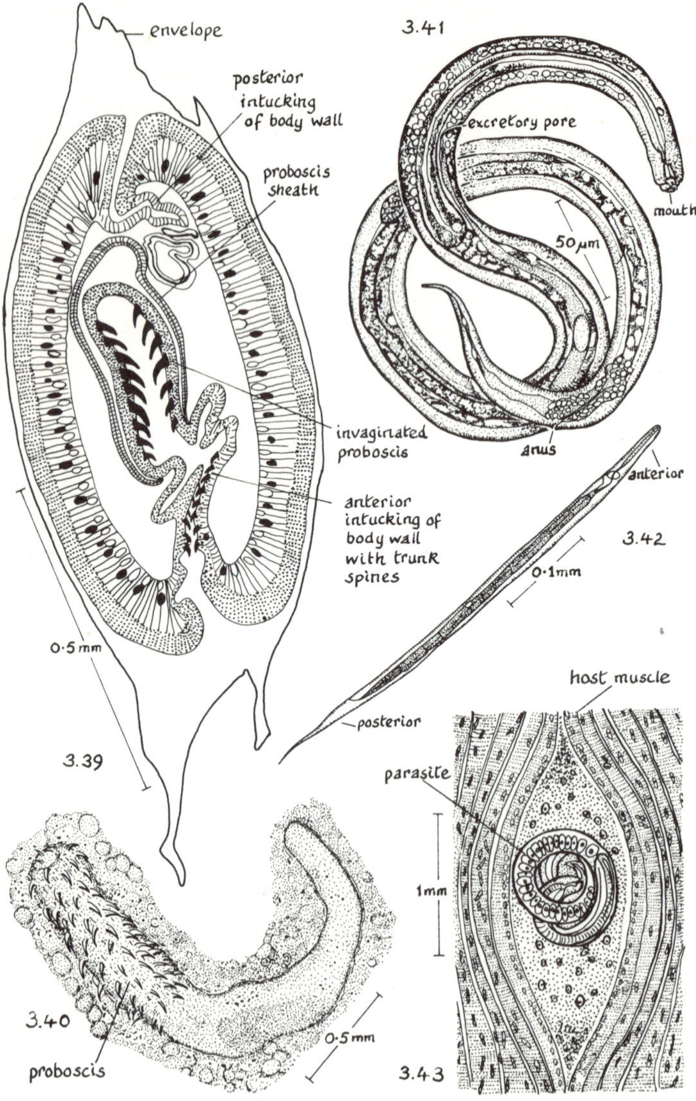


Figs. 3.39–3.43. Acanthocephalan and nematode infective stages. 3.39. Longitudinal section of a cystacanth of the acanthocephalan *Polymorphus minutus* (after Crompton, 1964). 3.40. Immature stage of the acanthocephalan *Leptorhynchoides thecatus* embedded in the peritoneum of a transport host (after Van Cleave, 1920, *J. Parasit.*, **6**, 167). 3.41. Infective third-stage larvae of *Ancylostoma* sp. (after Nichols, 1956, *J. Parasit.*, **42**, 363). 3.42. Third-stage larva (exsheathed) of *Haemonchus contortus* (after Dickmans and Andrews, 1933, *Trans Am. microsc. Soc.*, **52**, 1). 3.43. Larva of *Trichinella spiralis* encysted in mammalian muscle (after Faust, Russell and Jung, 1970. *Clinical Parasitology*, 8th edn.).

uninfected amphipods was studied in the laboratory with a light–dark choice acquarium. Uninfected amphipods were found to spend nearly all their time in the darker and deeper water. If the water surface was disturbed when an uninfected amphipod had reached the surface, the animal immediately dived for the refuge of the deep water. Infected *Gammarus*, however, displayed significantly different behaviour. They preferred to stay at the surface and reacted by clinging to bits of vegetation when the water was disturbed. Surface weed and floating vegetation form the bulk of the diet of a dabbling duck and the altered behaviour of *Gammarus lacustris* infected with *P. paradoxus* will almost certainly increase the chance of ducks acquiring the parasite. The change in the amphipod's behaviour seems to coincide with the formation of the cystacanth stage of *P. paradoxus*, which is similar in morphology to that of *P. minutus* (fig. 3.39). There would be a serious disadvantage for the survival of the parasite if the behavioural changes of the host occurred before the parasite was infective to ducks. The mechanism behind these changes is not yet

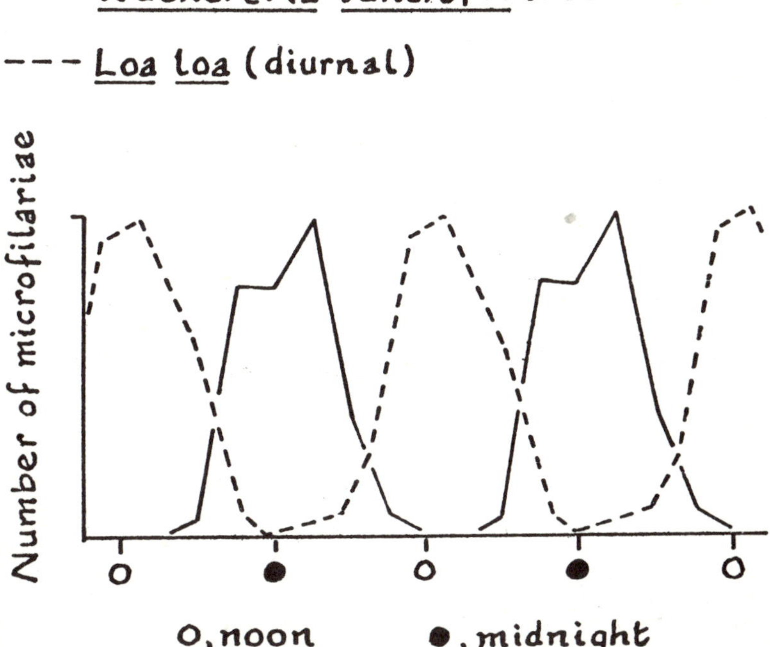


Fig. 3.44. Different patterns in the periodicity of occurrence of microfilariae in the circulating blood of man (after Kennedy, 1975).

known, since the presence of one or a few cystacanths in the amphipod's body cavity does not cause any obvious physical damage.

### 3.2.4. *Behaviour of adult helminths*

The egg-laying behaviour of adult nematodes may also increase the chances of successful transmission between hosts. Female thunder-worms, *Mermis nigrescens*, climb out of the soil and lay their eggs at the tips of grass shoots and on other plants. The eggshell is extended at each end to form a byssus or attachment device which ensures its adherence to the type of vegetation eaten by the insect intermediate hosts (fig. 3.15). Gravid pinworms, *Enterobius vermicularis*, journey by night from the large intestine of man to deposit eggs (fig. 3.12) around the anus. The irritation accompanying this event leads to scratching, contamination of the fingers with eggs and their inevitable transport to the mouth of the same or another host. Mature guinea worms, *Dracunculus medinensis*, which may have been the fiery serpents that afflicted the children of Israel during their flight from Egypt, emigrate to the surface layers of the skin of the legs when the parasite is about to produce its live offspring. The worm releases potent lytic substances which dissolve the skin and enable it to discharge infective larvae directly into water, the environment of the intermediate hosts.

Many other examples of adaptations for transmission and dispersal could have been described. Some helminth eggs appear to mimic diatoms or simple aquatic plants (fig. 3.5), some cercariae swim in a manner which may deceive mosquito-eating fish into mistaking them for mosquito larvae, and certain digenean sporocysts containing infective cercariae may play a part in drawing the attention of potential definitive hosts to a succulent snail.

## 3.3. *Mechanisms of infection*

### 3.3.1. *Ectoparasitic helminths*

The infection of various fish by the oncomiracidia of monogeneans (see fig. 3.17) and by cercariae (fig. 3.29) of the unusual digenean *Transversotrema patialense* have been studied in considerable detail. About 20 seconds after the arrival of an oncomiracidium of *Entobdella soleae* on the surface of a suitable host fish, the ciliated coat (fig. 3.17) is lost and the invader assumes obligatory dependence on its host.

The evidence indicates that a complex attachment process occurs after the cercariae of *T. patialense* (fig. 3.29) and their fish hosts have come into contact. Under experimental conditions, the cercariae usually swim tail first in active bursts lasting for 2 or 3 seconds. Between active bursts, the cercariae sink head down like minute aquatic parachutes with the tail fins spread out and the arms (fig. 3.30) extended. If a cercaria strikes a suitable fish during its descent, the adhesive pads at the ends of the arms (fig. 3.30) stick to the host's skin. For a moment, the cercaria has the appearance of a miniature gymnast performing a handstand. The body of the cercaria now unfolds and bends forward so that the dorsal surface of the body lies against the skin of the fish. The cercarial body then twists over and the ventral sucker grips the host. The twisting action dislodges the adhesive arms, which become detached when the motile tail breaks away from the body.

These observations on the attachment of cercariae of *T. patialense* to the skin of fish, pose many intriguing questions which are relevant to other host–parasite relationships involving both ectoparasitism and skin penetration. For example, the adhesive pads on the cercarial arms of *T. patialense* appear to produce a glue, but the events leading to its discharge and the nature of its rapid setting properties between wet surfaces have still to be explained.

### 3.3.2. *Endoparasitic helminths and the oral route of infection*

Most species of endoparasitic helminth appear to enter both intermediate and definitive hosts by way of the host's mouth. The infective stages may be general contaminants of the host's environment or drinking water, or specific contaminants of the diets of herbivores, omnivores and carnivores and even of the milk on which suckling mammals depend. Larval stages of the nematodes *Strongyloides ratti* and *Ancylostoma caninum* are known to be ingested by new-born rats and dogs, respectively, during suckling.

Apart from possessing structural features which render them resistant to adverse environmental conditions, many infective stages tend to have a low metabolic rate, which must contribute to their survival for long periods. In considering the oral route of infection, it is important to appreciate that certain properties of the new environment, provided by the alimentary tract of the susceptible host, stimulate and activate the semi-dormant parasite to escape from enclosing shells or sheaths and membranes before the motility of the tract has carried the parasite past the anus and out of the host again. Clearly, lack of stimulation followed by a return to the environment is advantageous if an infective stage has been swallowed by an inappropriate host. Eggs of the acanthocephalan *Macracanthorhyn-*

*chus hirudinaceus*, from which acanthors (see fig. 3.22) escape in the intestine of various species of beetle, pass apparently unchanged through the alimentary canal of pigeons. In host–parasite relationships involving the alimentary tract of vertebrates, it is nearly always observed that a particular parasitic worm occupies a fairly precise site in the tract (see Chapter 4). The tapeworm *Hymenolepis microstoma* is usually confined to the bile duct of mice and the acanthocephalan *Polymorphus minutus* to a region about two-thirds of the distance along the length of the small intestine of ducks (table 4.1). Many factors affect the distribution of helminths in the alimentary tract of vertebrates, but if some regions of the tract are unfavourable for the growth of certain parasites it is conceivable that the activating stimuli which are essential to infection may only exist and elicit a response in certain parts of the tract. The purpose of these general considerations is to stress that infection by the oral route is not necessarily a haphazard event.

The majority of investigations of infective stages have been carried out *in vitro* on parasites of vertebrates. Infective stages have been activated *in vitro* by exposing them to a variety of physical and chemical conditions. It has been found that a given infective stage responds to a certain range of temperatures, hydrogen ion concentrations, enzyme concentrations and so on. Activation can be judged to have occurred if major larval movements are seen or if previously inverted attachment organs become everted. Little is known, however, about how the activating conditions succeed in stimulating the infective stage, how the stimulus is received or whether exactly the same stimulating conditions operate *in vivo*. Some observations from experimental studies on the activation of the infective stages of various helminths which are ingested by vertebrates are summarized in table 3.2. Irrespective of whether or not the conditions which bring about activation *in vitro* exist in the alimentary tract, it is apparent from the information in the table that many infective stages are likely to be dependent on the host's digestive system for their release from the tissues of intermediate hosts. It is also likely that changes in the properties of cyst walls, egg shells and sheaths, which have been observed *in vitro* after the infective stages have been exposed to the activity of digestive enzymes (table 3.2), will occur in the vertebrate alimentary tract.

Much work has been done on the infection of ducks by the acanthocephalan *Polymorphus minutus* and a discussion of this host–parasite relationship will serve to illustrate various aspects of infection by the oral route. The references cited at the back of the book should be

TABLE 3.2. *Examples of factors which contribute to the activation and excystation* in vitro *of infective stages of worms in the vertebrate alimentary tract (after Lackie, 1975).*

| Parasitic worm | Infective stage[a] (definitive host) | Incubation conditions[b] |
|---|---|---|
| DIGENEA | | |
| *Cryptocotyle lingua* | Metacercaria in fish (seabirds) | 40 °C, pepsin, trypsin, bile salts (enhance) |
| *Fasciola hepatica* | Metacercaria on grass (sheep) | 39 °C, $CO_2$, reducing agent, bile |
| CESTODA | | |
| *Echinococcus granulosus* | Hydatid cyst—protoscolex in sheep (dogs) | 38 °C, pancreatic enzymes, bile salts (enhance) |
| *Hymenolepis diminuta* | Cysticercoid in beetles (rat) | 37 °C, pepsin (primes), trypsin, bile salts (activate) |
| ACANTHOCEPHALA | | |
| *Polymorphus minutus* (Table 3.3.) | Cystacanth in amphipod (duck) | 42 °C, bile salts (enhance) |
| NEMATODA | | |
| *Ascaris lumbricoides* | Egg (man, pig) | 37 °C, 5% $CO_2$, reducing agent |
| *Haemonchus contortus*[c] | Third-stage larva on grass (sheep) | (1) 37 °C, $CO_2$, $H_2CO_3$, reducing agent<br>(2) 40 °C, $CO_2$, sodium borate |

[a] Details of the morphology of infective stages are shown in the figures for this chapter.
[b] It is assumed that a suitable liquid medium and hydrogen ion concentration have been used.
[c] Activation and exsheathment (8.5) of larvae of this species have been achieved *in vitro* by means of different conditions.

consulted for examples involving other species of helminth in both invertebrate and vertebrate hosts. In nature, ducks acquire *P. minutus* by swallowing amphipod crustaceans in which the parasite has developed to the cystacanth stage (fig. 3.39). During development in the intermediate host, the anterior and posterior portions of the parasite become withdrawn into the middle portion of the body. These introversions result in the parasite's tissues forming a hard object occupying a small volume. The smallness and hardness of the cystacanth of *P. minutus* is not representative of all acanthocephalan cystacanths; in *P. minutus* the structure of the cystacanth appears to be a protective adaptation for withstanding the pressures and shearing forces generated in the muscular ventriculus (gizzard) of the duck.

Some results from a study of the process of infection of ducklings with *P. minutus* are given in table 3.3. Ducklings of the same sex and general age and the same nutritional status were fed known numbers of cystacanths in the intermediate host, *Gammarus pulex*. The fate of the parasite was recorded when the ducklings were examined at autopsy at known time intervals after the *Gammarus* had been swallowed. Throughout the study, the criterion used for determining the activation of a cystacanth was the eversion of the proboscis or anterior part of the body of the parasite. No cystacanths showed any signs of activation until they had been in the duck's alimentary tract for 25 minutes or longer (table 3.3). Activated parasites were found in the region extending from about two-thirds to three-quarters of the length of the small intestine, which is the portion of the small intestine occupied by mature *P. minutus*. Parasites which had not been activated by the time they had passed this zone did not become activated. The cystacanths were freed from the intermediate host's tissue by the contractions of the ventriculus and, although a few crushed cystacanths were retrieved from the ventriculus, on no occasion were activated cystacanths found until they had been propelled out of the ventriculus into the small intestine. In further experiments, cystacanths which had already been dissected out of their intermediate hosts were introduced directly into the small intestine by means of surgical techniques. Activation occurred and more parasites were found to be established in their normal habitat in the small intestine than was the case when passage through the ventriculus was involved.

These observations on the activation of cystacanths of *P. minutus in vivo* were used to design a series of experiments *in vitro* in which

TABLE 3.3. *Observations on the start of the course of infection of ducklings with* Polymorphus minutus *(Acanthocephala) (after Lingard and Crompton, 1972).*

| Time after ingestion (min) | Number of ducks | Fate of the cystacanths in the hosts | | | |
|---|---|---|---|---|---|
| | | Number given | Number retrieved | Number activated[a] | Number established[b] |
| 20 | 9 | 103 | 94 | 0 | 0 |
| 25 | 9 | 108 | 106 | 14 | 7 |
| 40 | 9 | 100 | 90 | 23 | 17 |
| 60 | 8 | 94 | 83 | 46 | 42 |
| 90 | 7 | 70 | 63 | 31 | 22 |

[a] Activation is defined as the eversion of any part of the anterior body or proboscis (fig. 3.39).

[b] Establishment is the attachment of the parasite to the intestinal wall.

cystacanths were exposed to varying conditions of temperature, hydrogen ion concentration and other factors (figs. 3.45–3.48). It was found that in a balanced salt solution, the optimum temperature for activation was 42 to 44 °C (fig. 3.45) at a pH of about 7.0 (fig. 3.46). An enhancement of activation rate occurred if the cystacanths were incubated for a few minutes in solutions of duck bile at physiological concentrations. Subsequent work traced this enhancing effect to chromatographically pure bile salts such as sodium taurocholate (fig. 3.47). The osmotic pressure of the surrounding medium also had an effect on activation as assessed in terms of proboscis eversion (fig. 3.39). Surgical transplantation of the artificially activated parasites into ducks demonstrated that the parasites had not lost their capacity to grow and develop in their natural hosts. The conditions for activation of cystacanths of *P. minutus in vitro* are not unlike those which have been found to exist in the alimentary tract of ducks. In the duck's ventriculus, the pH is usually below 4.0 and, in the light of the results in the *in vitro* studies, it is not surprising that activation does not occur there; if it did so, many cystacanths might be damaged. The enhancing effect of the bile salts is equally interesting and significant. Material passes rapidly along the alimentary tract of a duck and will normally arrive in the region occupied by *P. minutus* within 25–30 minutes of leaving the ventriculus. It can be seen from fig. 3.47 that the enhancing effect of bile appears to increase the chances of the parasite having an everted attachment organ by the time it has been carried to its habitat.

Bile salts have been known for a long time to contribute to the infection mechanisms of several species of helminth (table 3.2) and in some cases their participation appears to be obligatory. In digestion, bile salts function as detergents and are responsible for converting fat into soluble mixed micelles. In infection mechanisms, however, the role of bile salts is undetermined, but they could have three main effects: (*a*) initiation of permeability changes in membranes, (*b*) stimulation of increased muscular activity by the parasite and (*c*) enhancement of the activity of the host's digestive enzymes. Each or all of these effects could be important for the activation and release of semi-dormant parasites from egg shells, encapsulating tissues or cysts.

### 3.3.3. *Endoparasitic helminths and the cutaneous route of infection*

The miracidia and cercariae of many species of digenean fluke (figs. 3.18–3.20, 3.26–3.28) and the third-stage larvae of certain species of nematode (fig. 3.41) provide examples of infective stages which actively penetrate the skins and cuticles of their hosts in order to become established. Filarial nematodes also penetrate the host's skin, but the process is largely passive and is dependent on the mouthparts of blood-sucking flies.

The miracidia of *Fasciola*, the common liver fluke, are adapted to penetrate the skin of the snail *Lymnaea truncatula*. The structure of the surface which must be penetrated consists of mucus, columnar epithelial cells and a zone of loosely arranged muscles, gland cells and connective tissue. During penetration, the first phase of the metamorphosis of the miracidium of *Fasciola* into the sporocyst stage occurs. Early attachment of the miracidia to the exposed surfaces of the snail is often weak and many miracidia fail to attach firmly. Those which succeed in gripping the host's skin can be seen to be held by tiny cup-like suckers which have formed at the anterior end. The body of the attached miracidium begins to pulsate, and secretions are discharged from the various glands (see fig. 3.18). Within about 10 minutes of attachment, the snail's surface layers have been dissolved, presumably as a result of the miracidial secretions, and the parasite can be found to have penetrated as far as the connective tissue. This degree of penetration is accompanied by the shedding of the miracidial ciliated epithelium (see figs. 3.18 and 3.19), and by the time the parasite is completely enclosed by host tissue it has lost all its cilia. The parasite may now be regarded as a young sporocyst.

This description of miracidial penetration probably applies to many species of fluke. *Philophthalmus megalurus* is an interesting exception, however, because its miracidium already contains a sporocyst when the egg hatches in water. About half of the body of the miracidium penetrates into the tissues and then the sporocyst wriggles out of the miracidium and on into the host's tissues while the remnants of the miracidium drop off the snail and die. Some miracidia, for example those of *Dicrocoelium dendriticum*, do not escape from the eggshells until the egg has been swallowed by the appropriate species of snail. These miracidia are adapted to penetrate intestinal epithelial cells, as are the hexacanth larvae (oncospheres) and procercoids of many cestodes (figs. 3.21, 3.31), the acanthors of acanthocephalans (fig. 3.22) and the larval stages of certain nematodes.

The medical importance of the three highly pathogenic species of *Schistosoma* has prompted many studies of cercarial penetration of mammalian skin. Some details of the morphology and structure of skin are shown in fig. 3.49. Several studies have been made of the penetration of cercariae into rodent skin, which differs in several respects from that of man, the stratum corneum being proportionately thinner. The thickest skin in man is found on the soles of the feet and

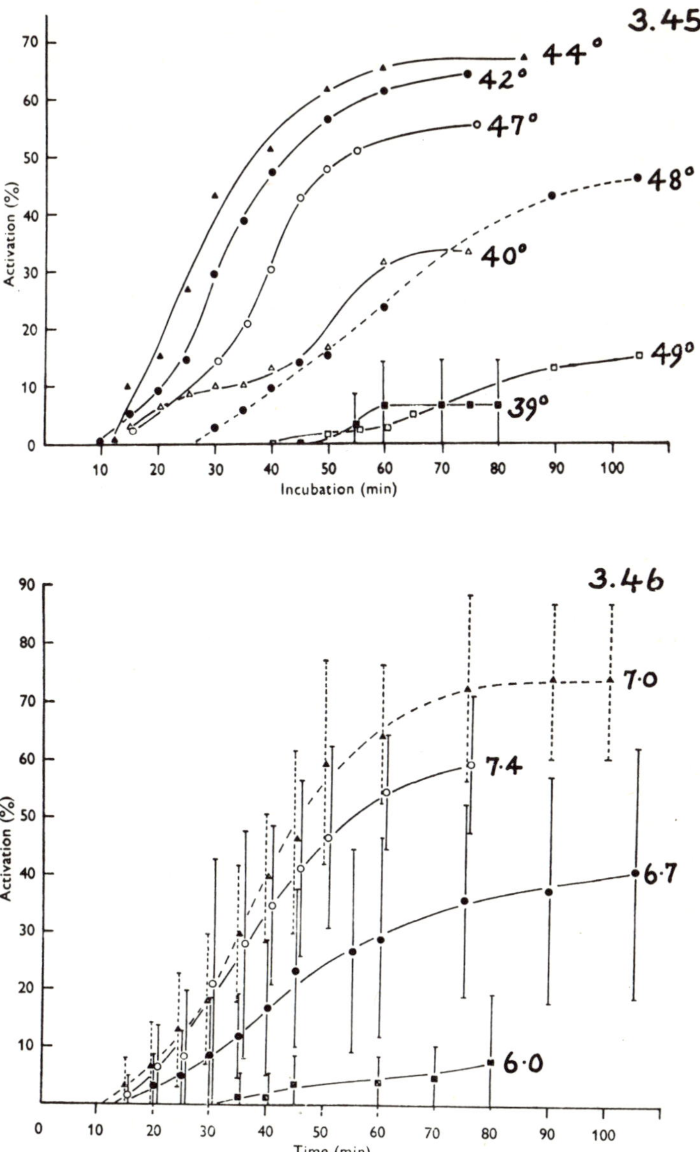


Figs. 3.45–3.48. Observations on the activation of cystacanths of *Polymorphus minutus* (Acanthocephala) *in vitro* (from Lackie, 1974, *Parasitology*, **68**, 135). 3.45. The effect of temperature (°C) on activation. 3.46. The effect of hydrogen ion concentration on activation. 3.47. The effect of different concentrations of bile salt (sodium taurocholate =NaTC) on activation (BSS=balanced salt solution). 3.48. The effect of osmotic pressure on activation. Osmolarity of solutions expressed as equivalent to mmol $l^{-1}$ NaCl. Bars show standard deviations in all figures.

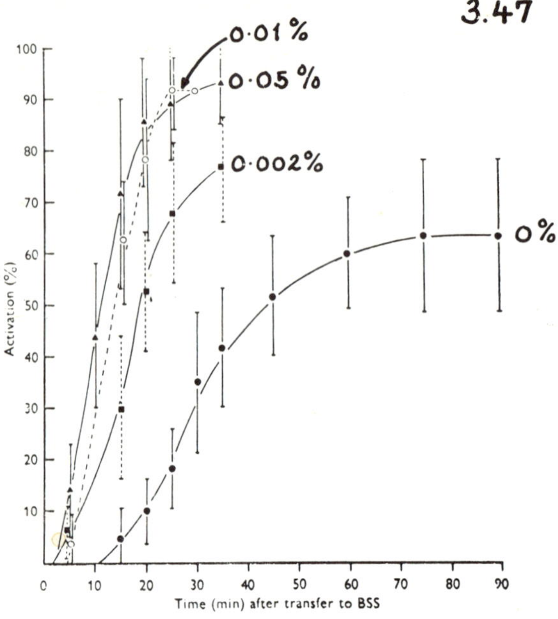
3.47
0·01 %
0·05 %
0·002%
0%
Activation (%)
Time (min) after transfer to BSS

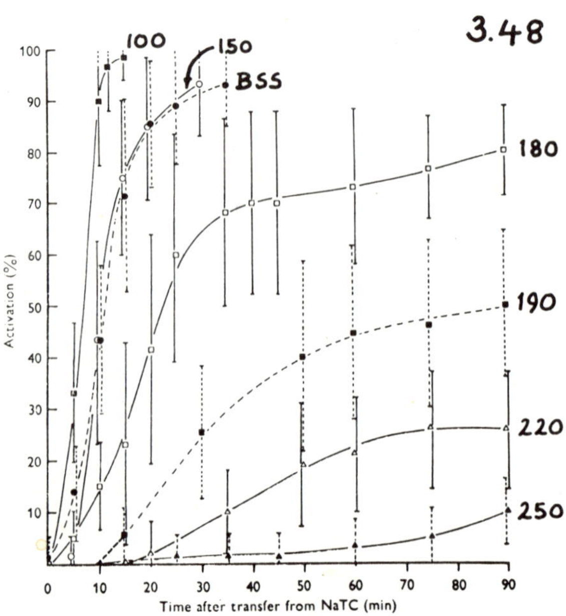
3.48
100
150
BSS
180
190
220
250
Activation (%)
Time after transfer from NaTC (min)

the palms of the hands; these may be the regions that are most frequently exposed to attack by cercariae or hookworm larvae.

In laboratory investigations, cercariae of *Schistosoma* seem to explore the skin surface for entry sites. Wrinkle crevices and hair projections appear to be the most favoured places for entry. The cercariae then secrete adhesive material from their gland cells (fig. 3.27) and become anchored perpendicularly to the surface of the skin. By the combined effects of muscular activity and further secretions, the stratum corneum is pierced and the cercarial tails fall away. The parasites are now known as schistosomula, and they release more secretions after a resting period. This bout of secretory activity is assumed to soften the deeper skin tissues, and the schistosomula move parallel to the basement membrane until they enter a sebaceous gland, which forms a natural route into the dermis. Once in the dermis of susceptible hosts, the schistosomula move efficiently at speeds varying from about 20 to 50 μm per minute in the skin of five-day-old rats. Gradually the parasites gain entry to the vascular system, in which they reach the liver and eventually the abdominal blood vessels.

There is now general agreement that the secretions of the cercariae of *Schistosoma* spp. are important for penetration of the skin. These secretions not only alter the properties of skin tissues, but also degrade

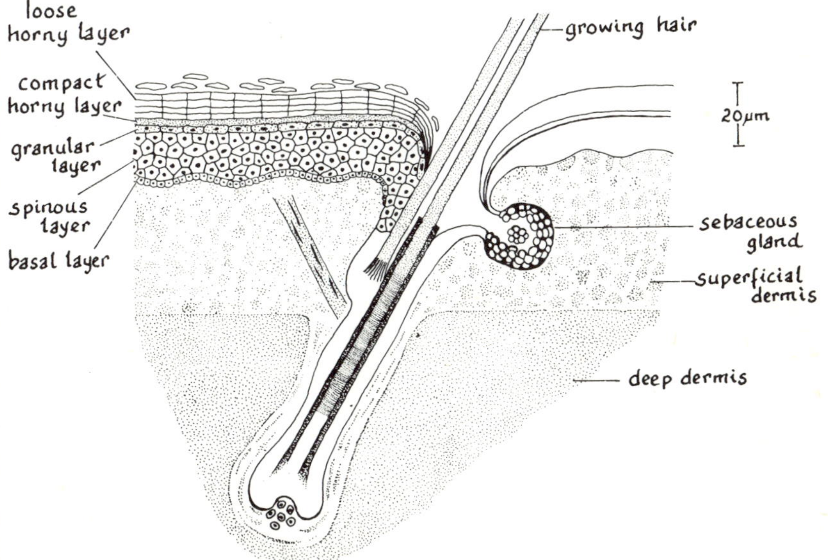


Fig. 3.49. The mammalian epidermis (after Spearman, 1973, *The Integument*).

hyaluronic acid, streptococcal capsules, heparin, mucopolysaccharide, collagen, elastin, polypeptides, casein and haemoglobin. The cercariae of other species of digenean fluke, however, penetrate their hosts by mainly mechanical means. The cercariae of *Plagiorchis megalorchis* (fig. 3.26) are equipped with a stylet which is used to make a slit in the cuticle of the midge larva to which a cercaria has attached. The cercaria then crawls through the slit into the host's body cavity. The whole process takes from about 2–13 minutes and the tail is usually lost during penetration.

In contrast to the penetrative mechanisms of schistosome cercariae, the third-stage larvae of hookworms (fig. 3.41) and related nematodes appear to rely mainly on mechanical rather than chemical processes. Evidence for the involvement of histolytic secretions is at present questionable and unconvincing. The third-stage larvae of *Nippostrongylus* may spend an hour on the surface of rat skin before beginning to burrow through into the tissues. The larvae appear to select their point of entry, and surface moisture appears to be important in enabling them to obtain an adequate purchase for the thrust of burrowing. Penetration of mouse skin may be achieved within 5 minutes by larvae of *Nippostrongylus*. Although infections of hookworm are usually assumed to start through penetration of the skin, the results of some studies indicate that many more worms from a given dose become established if the infective third-stage larvae are swallowed (table 3.4).

TABLE 3.4. *Infectivity of* Uncinaria stenocephala *larvae (species of canine hookworm) measured in susceptible pups by necropsy worm burdens after infection by various routes with 1000 larvae (from Miller, 1971,* Adv. Parasit., **9**, *153).*

| Route of infection | Number of of pups | Mean worm burdens |
|---|---|---|
| Larvae placed on skin | 4 | 6 |
| Larvae inoculated subcutaneously | 4 | 5 |
| Larvae inoculated intravenously | 4 | 152 |
| Larvae deposited in mouth | 3 | 469 |
| Larvae administered orally in gelatin capsules | 2 | 433 |

## 3.4. *Factors affecting transmission and infection*

Many ecological factors in the environments of vectors and of intermediate and definitive hosts influence transmission. Similarly, ecological factors will affect the activities and numbers of free infective stages. The number of infective stages available for transmission, whether they be free or dependent on some other agent, will be governed in part by the nature of the host–parasite relationship at the time of their release. Every aspect of a host–parasite relationship is affected by the pedigree, virulence and pathogenicity of the parasite and by the age, sex, and pedigree of the host together with its nutritional, physiological and immunological status. Evidence in support of this claim is to be found throughout this book.

# 4. Distribution of worms in their hosts

Parasitic worms are usually to be found in precise sites or microhabitats on or in their hosts. This generalization seems to apply to all the developmental stages of a parasite, irrespective of the status of its host. For example, the filarial nematode *Dirofilaria aethiops* inhabits at least four sites during its development in monkeys and mosquitoes. The adult worms live in the connective tissue of the monkey's thigh muscles, and the microfilariae live in the monkey's blood until they are ingested by mosquitoes. The worms then continue their development in the thoracic muscles of the mosquito before transferring to the salivary glands, whence they are discharged back into monkeys. In this chapter, an ecological approach is adopted in an attempt to study the distribution of worms in their habitats within their hosts. The habitat concept is always difficult to explain; every biologist knows what it is yet many might be hard pressed to propose an acceptable definition, especially when confronted with fixing the bounds of a particular organism's habitat. It is often accepted, however, that a habitat possesses a certain uniformity with respect to some quality which the ecologist decides is important for his study. For example, the littoral zone of the sea shore may be given the status of a habitat because all its features are influenced by the tides. Similarly, the physiological function of an organ system within the host may be considered as providing the necessary uniformity of a habitat. In this chapter most emphasis is given to the distribution of helminths in vertebrate definitive hosts.

## 4.1. *Distribution of worms in definitive hosts*

Some idea of the sites of helminths in the habitats occurring in definitive vertebrate hosts is given in table 4.1 and figs. 4.1–4.5. The sites listed are those in which the worms attain maturity. Careful scrutiny of the extensive available literature would support the conclusion drawn from the table that cestodes and acanthocephalans are usually confined to the small intestine, that monogeneans and digeneans, with the exception of blood flukes, are nearly always associated with epithelial cells, and that nematodes are to be found in almost every organ system of the vertebrate body. The distribution no doubt depends on the places in the host where the appropriate shelter and resources for a particular worm are to be found. Food is likely to be a major resource, and the varied distribution of nematodes in definitive hosts, compared with that of cestodes and acanthocephalans, may be associated with the fact that nematodes have retained a functional alimentary tract during their evolution and thus have many more diets available to them. The small size of many species of nematode may have facilitated their colonization of the many potential micro-habitats in the vertebrate body. Digenean flukes are also small and have an alimentary tract, but they seem to have become specialized for exploitation of the nutrients liberated during their browsing on the epithelial cells of skin surfaces, duct linings and the alimentary tract.

The vertebrate alimentary tract is a fascinating habitat for study. During digestion, many processes occur simultaneously in the alimentary canal, with the result that different concentrations of enzymes, bile salts and other molecules prevail at different places along the length of the tract. Thus, different environmental conditions can be demonstrated to exist and it is attractive to suggest that the distribution of worms in the tract, or in any other organ system, is related to the conditions found therein. There is still little unequivocal evidence in support of this point of view. Some intestinal worms must experience different environmental conditions at their anterior and posterior ends. The acanthocephalan *Neoechinorhynchus topsei* extends for the entire length of the small and large intestine of host mango fish. During digestion, the anterior and posterior parts of the strobila of a large tapeworm such as *Diphyllobothrium latum*, which may be 9 m long, may well experience different physicochemical conditions. The functions of the anterior and posterior regions of the strobila are different, and it may be that conditions in the anterior part of the host's tract favour the generation of proglottides more than the development of eggs.

*Hymenolepis microstoma* is a much smaller tapeworm than *D. latum*, but features of its distribution are equally interesting. Mice are its typical hosts, and it attaches to the wall of the bile duct and extends into the duodenum (table 4.1). The tapeworm will also infect hamsters and rats, and in a series of experimental infections the number of worms attached to the duodenum was found to be greater in rats than in hamsters and greater in hamsters than in mice. Forty-

TABLE 4.1. *The distribution of some adult parasitic worms in their definitive hosts.*

| Parasitic worm | Host | Usual site (microhabitat) |
|---|---|---|
| SKIN | | |
| M. *Entobdella soleae* | f. *Solea solea* (common sole) | Skin of lower (white) surface |
| D. *Transversotrema patialense* | f. *Brachydanio rerio* (zebra fish) | Sub-scale recesses of mid-flank |
| GILLS AND LUNGS | | |
| M. *Diclidophora merlangi* | f. *Gadus merlangus* (whiting) | First gill arch |
| D. *Haematoloechus medioplexus* | a. *Rana pipiens* (adult frog) | Attached to wall of lungs |
| D. *Paragonimus westermani* | m. Domestic cat | In cysts in pulmonary tissue |
| N. *Dictyocaulus viviparus* | m. Domestic cattle | Bronchial tree |
| BODY CAVITIES | | |
| N. *Litomosoides carinii* | m. *Sigmodon hispidus litoralis* (cotton rat) | Pleural cavity |
| MUSCULATURE | | |
| N. *Dirofilaria aethiops* | m. *Cercopithecus aethiops* (monkey) | Connective tissue of thigh muscles |
| LIVER AND DIGESTIVE ORGANS | | |
| D. *Eurytrema vulpis* | m. *Vulpes vulpes* (fox) | Pancreatic ducts |
| D. *Fasciola hepatica* | m. Domestic sheep and laboratory mouse | Biliary system |
| N. *Capillaria hepatica* | m. Rodents | Hepatic tissue |
| ALIMENTARY TRACT | | |
| D. *Apatemon gracilis minor* | b. Domestic duck | Anterior third of small intestine |
| D. *Psilostomum ondatrae* | b. Domestic fowl | Mucosa of proventriculus |
| D. *Renifer aniarum* | r. *Natrix sipedon* (water snake) | Mouth cavity |
| C. *Echinococcus granulosus* | m. Domestic dog | Between villi in duodenum |
| C. *Hymenolepis diminuta* | m. Laboratory rat | Small intestine (circadian migration) |
| C. *Hymenolepis microstoma* | m. Laboratory mouse | Attached to bile duct, extends into duodenum |
| C. *Moniezia expansa* | m. Domestic sheep | Small intestine |

| | | |
|---|---|---|
| C. *Phyllobothrium piriei* | f. *Raja naevus* (ray) | Posterior-facing surfaces of tiers in spiral valve |
| C. *Raillietina cesticillus* | b. Domestic fowl | Anterior small intestine |
| A. *Moniliformis dubius* | m. Laboratory rat | Anterior half of small intestine |
| A. *Polymorphus minutus* | b. Domestic duck | Posterior half of small intestine |
| N. *Ascaris lumbricoides* | m. Domestic pig | Anterior half of small intestine |
| N. *Haemonchus contortus* | m. Domestic sheep | Mucosa of abomasum |
| N. *Heterakis gallinarum* | b. Domestic fowl | Distal lumen of caeca |
| N. *Nippostrongylus brasiliensis* | m. Laboratory rat | Mucosa of anterior small intestine |
| N. *Spirocerca lupi* | m. Domestic dog | Wall of oesophagus |
| N. *Tachygonetria* spp. | r. *Testudo graeca* (tortoise) | Lumen of large intestine |
| N. *Trichuris trichiura* | m. Man | Associated with wall of large intestine |
| URINOGENITAL SYSTEM | | |
| M. *Polystoma integerrimum* | a. *Rana temporaria* (frog) | Attached to bladder wall |
| D. *Gorgodera amplicava* | a. *Rana palustris* (frog) | Bladder and urinogenital ducts |
| D. *Prosthogonimus macrorchis* | b. Female domestic fowl | Oviducts |
| N. *Dioctophyma renale* | m. *Mustela vison* (mink) | Kidney |
| N. *Trichosomoides crassicauda* | m. Laboratory rat | Bladder |
| SENSORY AND NERVOUS SYSTEMS | | |
| D. *Halipegus eccentricus* | a. *Rana pipiens* (frog) | Eustachian tubes (ears) |
| N. *Oxyspirura mansoni* | b. Domestic fowl | Beneath nictating membrane (eyes) |
| VASCULAR AND LYMPHATIC SYSTEMS | | |
| D. *Sanguinicola kalmathensis* | f. *Salmo clarkii henshawi* (cutthroat trout) | Efferent renal vein |
| D. *Schistosoma mansoni* | m. Laboratory mouse | Mesenteric veins |
| N. *Angiostrongylus cantonensis* | m. Laboratory rat | Pulmonary arteries |
| N. *Dirofilaria immitis* | m. Domestic dog | Right ventricle and pulmonary arteries |
| N. *Wuchereria bancrofti* | m. Man | Lymphatic vessels and glands |

A, Acanthocephala; C, Cestoda; D, Digenea; M, Monogenea; N, Nematoda.
a, Amphibian; b, Bird; f, Fish; m, Mammal; r, Reptile.

two out of 116 infected rats harboured *H. microstoma* attached to the duodenum, whereas only 3 tapeworms were observed to be attached to the duodenum in a sample of 170 infected mice. The tapeworm *Schistocephalus solidus* is also unusual in having wide host specificity and varied distribution in experimental hosts. The sites which *S. solidus* occupies in three species of bird and two species of mammal are shown in fig. 4.1 and it is likely that the physicochemical conditions in these sites will differ.

Occasionally, a site of a worm in a host may only be habitable for a relatively brief period. Flukes of the genus *Prosthogonimus* live in the avian oviduct, which normally provides a suitable environment only during the breeding season. Man's need for food, however, has led to the domestication of the fowl and the provision of an almost permanent site for *P. marcrorchis* (table 4.1).

### 4.1.1. *Descriptions of sites occupied by worms*

Comment on the distribution of helminths should always be made with caution until the reliability of the primary observations has been

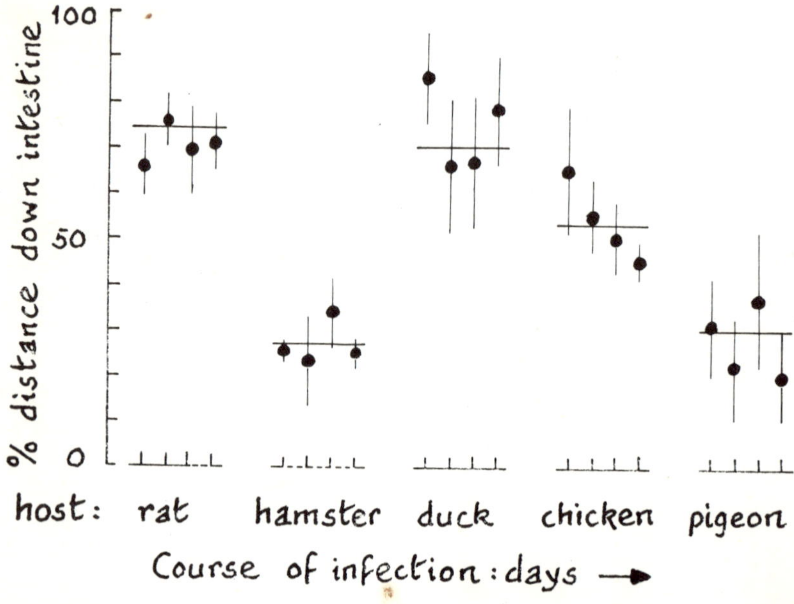


Fig. 4.1. The position of populations of *Schistocephalus solidus* (Cestoda) during the course of infection in the small intestine of different laboratory hosts. The closed circles represent the mean positions of worms and the vertical lines represent standard deviations. The horizontal lines indicate the mean positions of all the worms in their host (after McCaig and Hopkins, 1963, *Exptl Parasit.*, **13**, 273).

assessed. Most information is available about the distribution of worms in the alimentary tract. Ideally, the description of an alimentary site should include details about (*a*) the worm's linear and radial distribution, (*b*) the length of time which passed between the death of a host and finding the worms, (*c*) the time of day when the search was made, (*d*) the stage of digestion in progress on the death of the host, (*e*) the season of the year when the worms were observed, (*f*) the worm's reproductive and developmental state and (*g*) observations on the numbers of worms and other parasites present in the tract. This list has been compiled with the wisdom of hindsight, but the following examples will emphasize that each item is important if accurate information is to be obtained. Although these examples are taken from alimentary host–parasite relationships, they apply in principle to all aspects of the distribution of parasites in hosts.

In the alimentary tract, linear distribution is probably best expressed in terms of percentage distance from an anatomical reference point such as the pylorus (fig. 4.2). Detailed information about the anatomy, histology and physiology of the organ systems of a host is an essential part of any study of parasites and is one of the features which make parasitology so attractive and stimulating for the student. Information about the radial distribution also helps to define a worm's site when it inhabits a tube such as the alimentary canal and is small relative to the diameter of the tube (fig. 4.3). Furthermore, the physicochemical conditions across the lumen of the tract are not the same. A considerable oxygen tension exists close to the mucosa, whereas virtually no oxygen can be detected in the middle of the lumen. The movements of the intestinal contents, which contain suspended solids and long chain molecules in solution, exhibit plug flow and material near the walls of the tube will move with low velocity. The region close to the villi of the small intestine has been called the paramucosal lumen on account of its special features and it is important to know which species of worm live there. Worms may also penetrate to a characteristic depth in an organ or occupy a particular layer of the intestinal wall.

*Post mortem* changes occur in hosts, and these may contribute to the apparent distribution of worms. The nematode *Trichostrongylus axei* occurs in the stomach wall of freshly killed rabbits, but the worms are recovered from the lumen of the stomach when dead hosts are left for some hours before autopsy. A record of the time of day when the host was killed should be included in the description of a site because certain helminths are known to migrate in their host's tract. The cestode *Hymenolepis* living in laboratory rats maintained

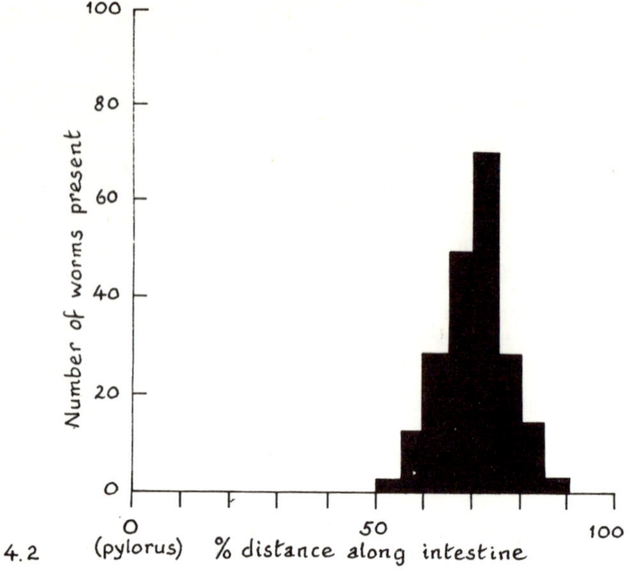


Figs. 4.2 and 4.3. Observations on the distribution of parasitic worms in their definitive hosts. 4.2. *Polymorphus minutus* (Acanthocephala) in domestic ducks (after Crompton and Harrison, 1965, *Parasitology*, **55**, 345). 4.3. Female worms of eight species of *Tachygonetria* (Nematoda) in the large intestine of tortoises (after Schad, 1963, *Nature, Lond.*, **198**, 404).

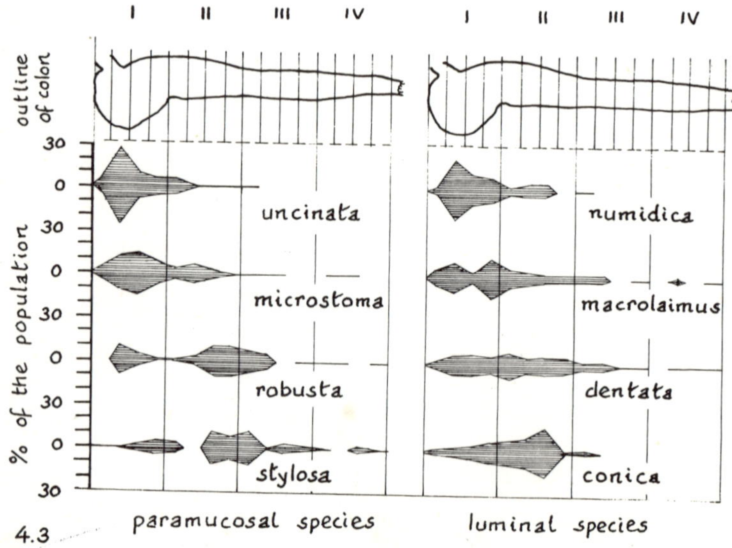

on a precise feeding routine displays a circadian migration (see Chapter 5) up and down the small intestine, and thus its site cannot be recorded with any more precision than 'small intestine' (table 4.1). If worms are influenced by the host's feeding routine, which must in turn affect the host's digestive physiology, the need to note the digestive and nutritional state of the host is self-evident.

The season of the year should also be included in the description of a site. This information may be of importance in studies of intestinal worms because it points to seasonal dietary changes or periods of fasting by the host. The digenean fluke *Podocotyle* sp. is known to live more anteriorly in the gut of the flounder *Platichthys flesus* in winter than it does in other seasons. Seasonal effects on distribution

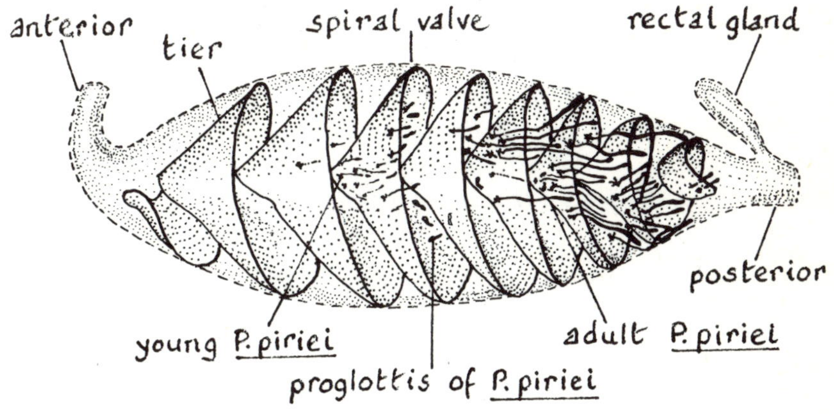


Fig. 4.4. The distribution of *Phyllobothrium piriei* (Cestoda) in the spiral valve of *Raja naevus* (after Williams, 1968, *Parasitology*, **58**, 929).

are observed not only with intestinal worms. In summer, the blood fluke *Sanguinicola inermis* inhabits the blood vessels of the gills of carp, but in winter the worms occur in the bulbus arteriosus, which is an enlargement of the ventral aorta near its exit from the heart. The season of the year may also give some clue to the reproductive state of a worm, since some worms, particularly those from poikilothermic hosts, show seasonal cycles of reproductivity. Information about reproductive development may be misleading if the age of the worms is not known. The cestode *Phyllobothrium piriei* lives in the spiral valve of elasmobranch fish (fig. 4.4). The larger cestodes are usually found attached to the tiers at the posterior end of the valve while the smaller individuals with less well-developed gonads, are found more anteriorly. Unless the age of the worms is available, however, there is no way of knowing whether the anterior worms are young specimens with predictably undeveloped gonads or whether they are older *P. piriei* whose gonads are developing more slowly because the optimal site in the posterior part of the spiral valve is fully occupied. The compactness of some of the sites of worms (table 4.1) justifies these regions being referred to as 'zones of optimal viability'. Evidence in support of this notion is provided by the observation that when large numbers of worms are present, those that are located at the fringe of the optimal zone tend to be smaller and less vigorous. Thus, when a site is described, information is needed about worm burden and about the other parasites present, since these may be potential competitors. Finally, information about the host's age and sex is important because these are two of the many host-mediated factors which may affect a population of worms and consequently the volume of space which is occupied in the habitat.

### 4.1.2. *Population effects on distribution*

The sites available for the establishment of worms in the various organ systems of a host are bound to be limited in terms of available space, and increase in the size of a population of worms is bound to result in excessive demands being put on environmental resources. The amount of available food and the number of worms dependent on it are often considered to give rise to 'crowding effects'. In a typical crowding effect, the worms are usually numerous, but showing signs of stunted growth and reduced fecundity, and often they may be occupying an extended site. In a duck, most individuals of *Polymorphus minutus* are usually found attached in the zone extending from about 65 to 80% of the distance along the small intestine from the pylorus (fig. 4.2). In a laboratory infection, 30 or more worms may be present in this region without any obvious signs of crowding. In a natural infection in a wild duck, however, several hundred *P. minutus* can be found packed into the posterior part of the small intestine. Many of these worms appear stunted, but it is not known whether the stunting stems from an initial pressure for space or from a shortage of other requirements. If space is the limiting resource, the over-crowded worms may interfere with each other's feeding activities and in this way be deprived of nutrients. Curiously, although *H. microstoma* shows many signs of a crowding effect in experimental infections in mice (table 4.2), the worm does not extend its site beyond the confined space of the bile duct until relatively large populations have become established. In other host–parasite relationships, a very different situation occurs, and very small populations of

TABLE 4.2. *Population density effect: experimental infections of* Hymenolepis microstoma *(Cestoda) in laboratory mice (after Jones and Tan, 1971).*

| Number of worms per mouse at autopsy | Mean worm length (mm) | Estimate of mean number of proglottides produced per worm per day | Estimate of mean number of eggs produced per worm per day | Estimate of mean number of eggs produced by population per day |
|---|---|---|---|---|
| 1 | 320 | 67 | 45 600 | 45 600 |
| 3 | 286 | 60 | 32 600 | 97 800 |
| 5 | 274 | 51 | 25 300 | 126 500 |
| 9 | 257 | 32 | 14 400 | 129 600 |
| 13 | 115 | 30 | 11 000 | 143 000 |
| 18 | 151 | 28 | 7700 | 138 600 |

worms are found even when ample space for several worms would appear to exist. For example, out of a sample of 62 cod fish infected with the tapeworm *Abothrium gadi*, 44 harboured only 1 tapeworm each (table 4.3), and the highest incidence of infection was in the biggest fish. There is no satisfactory explanation for these observations on *A. gadi*, nor for similar observations involving other host–parasite relationships. Presumably each of the cod fish that sheltered only one worm had eaten many more than one infected intermediate host. In contrast, enormous numbers of other species of helminth become established in other hosts and, although crowding effects probably occur and attachment sites become extended, restriction of population size is not always evident. As many as 15 000 specimens of the tapeworm *Hymenolepis spiralibursata* have been found in the small intestine of a wild mallard, over 100 000 specimens of the pinworm *Atractis dactyluris* have regularly been collected from the large intestine of tortoises, and about 200 000 specimens of the fluke *Nanophyetus salmincola* from the small intestine of a dog. This last species is a tiny worm which becomes almost completely buried

TABLE 4.3. *Cod infected with* Abothrium gadi *(Cestoda) grouped according to tapeworm population size (from Williams and Halvorsen, 1971.* Nor. J. Zool. **19**, *193).*

| *A. gadi* population size | 1 | 2 | 3 | 4 | 5 | 6 |
|---|---|---|---|---|---|---|
| Number of cod | 44 | 11 | 4 | 2 | 0 | 1 |
| Percentage of infected cod | 71 | 17.7 | 6.5 | 3.2 | 0 | 1.6 |

between the villi. Dogs acquire the infection by eating salmon, which may contain up to 40 000 metacercariae per gram of tissue.

### 4.1.3. *Interspecific effects of distribution*

Many observations have indicated that the distribution of a worm in its host may be affected by the presence of another species of worm or by other organisms in the same host. In three-spined sticklebacks, the sites of immature stages of the acanthocephalan *Neoechinorhynchus rutili* and adult stages of the tapeworm *Proteocephalus filicollis* were observed to be significantly different in concurrent infections. In single-species infections in sticklebacks, 99 tapeworms were recovered from the anterior half of the small intestine and 77 were in the posterior half, while in other sticklebacks 23 acanthocephalans were in the posterior half of the small intestine and 19 were in the rectum. In concurrent infections, nearly all the tapeworms were found in the anterior half of the small intestine and a greater number of the acanthocephalans was retrieved from the rectum. Although quantitative studies involving experimental infections with known numbers of tapeworms and acanthocephalans need to be carried out, it appears that in concurrent infections each species moves out of the part of its site where overlap occurs. Under experimental conditions, laboratory mice can become infected with the liver fluke *Fasciola* which reaches maturity in the common bile duct, and its presence has a striking effect on the distribution of *H. microstoma* (table 4.4). When mice infected with both species were examined at autopsy, nearly all the tapeworms had changed their attachment position from the wall of the bile duct, which was occupied by the flukes, to the duodenal mucosa. The tapeworms from the concurrent infections also weighed less than those from the single-species infections, and on average were fewer in number at the end of the experimental period (table 4.4). It is not known how the tapeworm becomes displaced from its site. Perhaps the fluke's excretory products contaminate the environment.

Changes in the distribution of blood flukes in rock fish from the Pacific coastal waters of North America were observed in concurrent infections. *Aporocotyle macfarlani* was always found in the afferent branchial arteries and sometimes in the chambers of the heart itself. *Psettarium sebastodorum* was found in the atrium and ventricle of the heart, but when both species of fluke were present in the same host, fewer *P. sebastodorum* were found in the ventricle and more were present in the atrium. The fluke *Haematoloechus medioplexus* lives firmly attached to the walls of the lungs of frogs (table 4.1).

Nematodes of the genus *Rhabdonema* are also common in the lungs of frogs, but some form of incompatibility appears to exist between *Haematoloechus* and *Rhabdonema* which may result in the fluke being confined to one lung and the nematode to the other in heavy concurrent infections. These shifts in distribution suggest that the worms may not be able to tolerate physical contact with each other. In the

TABLE 4.4. *Interspecific effects: experimental infections of* Fasciola hepatica *(Digenea) and* Hymenolepis microstoma *(Cestoda) in laboratory mice (after Lang, 1967).*

| | 56 male mice 22 weeks old | | |
|---|---|---|---|
| | Group I 24 mice | Group II 8 mice | Group III 24 mice |
| Day 0 | Dose of 5 cysticercoids per mouse | Dose of 5 cysticercoids per mouse | — |
| Day 25 | Dose of 2 metacercariae per mouse | — | Dose of 2 metacercariae per mouse |
| Day 85 (autopsy) | 1. 18 mice survived.<br>2. 45 out of 90 tapeworms were present, but many were attached to the duodenum and not the wall of the bile duct.<br>3. 32 out of 36 flukes were present, and all were in the bile duct. | 1. All mice survived.<br>2. 32 out of 40 tapeworms were present, and all were attached to the wall of the bile duct. | 1. 18 mice survived.<br>2. 28 out of 36 flukes were present, and all were in the bile duct. |

most extreme form, interspecific effects may result in the exclusion of one species of worm from a host which is already occupied by another species. For example, the tapeworm *Cittotaenia pectinata* normally occupies an anterior site in the small intestine of rabbits and *C. denticulata* occupies a posterior site. In a study involving many rabbits, the two species were not found in the same host even though their sites do not appear to overlap.

## 4.2. *Distribution of worms in intermediate hosts*

The sites in intermediate hosts occupied by the wide variety of developmental stage of worms have attracted less attention than the sites of their adult relatives, perhaps because intermediate hosts are often small and of less importance to man. Some information about the habitats of developing stages is summarized in table 4.5 and it

TABLE 4.5. *The distribution of some developmental stages of endoparasitic worms in intermediate hosts.*

| Stage | Common hosts | Common sites (microhabitats) |
|---|---|---|
| DIGENEA | | |
| Sporocyst (fig. 8.5) | Snails | Mantle, head and foot |
| Redia (fig. 8.6) | | Digestive gland and gonads |
| Metacercaria (figs. 3.36–3.38) | Leeches | Parenchymal tissue |
| | Molluscs | Gills, digestive gland and gonads |
| | Insects | Body cavity and muscles |
| | Crabs | Gills and muscles |
| | Fish | Skin and muscles |
| | Tadpoles | Tail (until metamorphosis) |
| CESTODA[a] | | |
| Procercoid (fig. 3.31) | Copepods | Body cavity |
| Plerocercoid (fig. 3.34)[b] | Teleost fish | Body cavity |
| Cysticercoid (fig. 3.32)[c] | Arthropods | Body cavity |
| Cysticercus (fig. 3.33)[d] | Mammals | Muscles |
| Hydatid cyst (fig. 3.35) | Mammals | Liver, lungs and other organs |
| ACANTHOCEPHALA | | |
| Acanthella (figs. 8.17–8.20) | Arthropods | Body cavity |
| Cystacanth (fig. 3.39) | | |
| NEMATODA (indirect cycles) | | |
| Filarial larvae (figs. 3.23–3.25) | Insects | Thoracic muscles |
| Spirurid larvae | Insects | Body tissues |

[a] The term 'metacestode' is often used to describe a stage or succession of stages which occur within intermediate hosts.

[b] In the Mazurian Lake area of Poland, local people have been observed to fry and eat plerocercoids obtained from local fish.

[c] *Hymenolepis nana*, a tapeworm from mice and men, usually develops with a direct life cycle. The eggs hatch in the host's duodenum and the oncospheres (fig. 8.9) penetrate the villi and develop into cysticercoids. The cysticercoids then break out of the duodenal villi and become established as young tapeworms in the posterior part of the small intestine.

[d] In a grim experiment in the middle of the last century, Küchenmeister fed cysticerci, in a meal of rice, vermicelli and black puddings, to a condemned murderer. On dissection of the cadaver, 48 hours after the execution, 10 young tapeworms were found and the biological significance of the cysticercus had been established.

appears that precise microhabitats may be identified for different species. For example, the mother sporocysts of the digenean fluke *Alaria arisaemoides* occupy the perioesophageal blood sinus of the snail host, while the daughter sporocysts inhabit the cavity surrounding the digestive gland. The daughter sporocysts of *Schistosoma*, however, develop within the digestive gland of the snail. Many metacercarial stages develop in secondary intermediate hosts into which they penetrate as cercariae. The metacercariae are usually found near the place of penetration, and in amphibian tadpoles the tail seems to be most vulnerable to cercarial attack. The metamorphosis of the tadpole into the frog involves the loss of the tail, and before development into the metacercarial stage is completed, the parasites have been observed to move into the region of the host's thighs. Other metacercariae have even more restricted microhabitats in secondary intermediate hosts. The metacercariae of flukes of the genus *Diplostomum* often inhabit the eye lens of fish and those of *Dicrocoelium dendriticum* frequently live in the suboesophageal ganglia of ants. It is to be expected that as many factors as affect the distribution of worms in definitive hosts will influence the distribution of their developing stages in the intermediate hosts.

## 4.3 *Emigration during development and site selection*

Parasitic worms do not always reach, immediately upon entry, those sites in a host where they will spend most time. Hookworms and blood flukes (table 4.6) inhabit sites a relatively long distance away from the skin. The juvenile hookworms and schistosomula must emigrate from the subcutaneous layers of the host to the alimentary tract and abdominal blood vessels respectively. Further examples of the variety of emigrations undertaken by parasitic worms in vertebrate hosts are given in table 4.6. Some salient features of emigrations are clearly demonstrated by the species listed in the table. Some emigrations are brief (*Oxyspirura mansoni*) and others are extended in time (*Spirocerca lupi*). Consideration of the time factor suggests that some worms may need to reach the appropriate site before they use up their endogenous reserves, while others may need to feed in a series of transient sites before becoming established in a permanent place. Some worms (*Fasciola*) appear to eat their way to their sites, whereas others (*Dioctophyma renale*) may dissolve the tissues through which they tunnel. The fact that the permanent sites are often very precise in their location (table 4.1) suggests that marked site specificity exists for many species of nematode and it is almost impossible to study emigrations and the distribution of worms in their hosts without reflecting that site selection may involve the directed behaviour of the worms.

TABLE 4.6. *Examples of emigrations undertaken by parasitic worms in vertebrate hosts. Names of hosts and sites where adulthood is attained are given in table 4.1 (after Crompton, 1976).*

| Parasitic worm | Emigration |
|---|---|
| MONOGENEA | |
| *Entobdella soleae* | Oncomiracidia invade upper surface of host, young flukes gather round head region before crawling over skin to sites on lower surface. |
| *Polystoma integerrimum* | Larvae enter gill chambers of tadpole and when metamorphosis begins, larvae leave gill chambers at night, crawl over skin and pass through cloaca into bladder. |
| DIGENEA | |
| *Fasciola hepatica* | After excystation in small intestine of mouse, young flukes tunnel through intestinal wall into body cavity. Next they penetrate liver and reside for some weeks in hepatic tissue before invading biliary system. |
| *Halipegus eccentricus* | Young flukes remain with little development at cardiac end of stomach of tadpoles in which metacercariae excyst. At metamorphosis, flukes move out of stomach, up oesophagus, across mouth and into eustachian tubes. |
| *Schistosoma mansoni* | After penetration of the skin, schistosomula enter veins and lymphatics to reach right side of heart and lungs before entering liver. Mature flukes leave liver and move into mesenteric veins. |
| CESTODA | |
| *Echinococcus granulosus* | Oncospheres bore into tissues of intestinal villi. In non-ruminant intermediate hosts, they tend to enter venules and reach liver. In ruminant intermediate hosts, they tend to enter lacteals and reach lungs. |
| *Hymenolepis microstoma* | Cysticercoids excyst in anterior small intestine where young tapeworms are found. After 4 days, most worms have become attached to wall of bile duct while extending into duodenum. |

TABLE 4.6.—*continued*

| Parasitic worm | Emigration |
|---|---|
| ACANTHOCEPHALA | |
| *Moniliformis dubius* | Cystacanths are activated in posterior small intestine where young worms become attached. By time worms are 4 weeks old, they are found attached to wall of anterior small intestine. |
| NEMATODA | |
| *Angiostrongylus cantonensis* | After ingestion, third-stage larvae penetrate intestinal wall and most each liver within an hour. They enter posterior vena cava, reach right atrium of heart, then lungs before entering main arterial circulation. Larvae are then dispersed through body. Many enter CNS where third moult occurs 5 days post infection. Fourth moult occurs 10 days post infection, worms enter cerebral veins and gain access to pulmonary arterial system. |
| *Dioctophyma renale* | After ingestion, larvae assumed to penetrate duodenal wall and cross abdominal cavity at point where duodenum is nearest to right kidney. |
| *Nippostrongylus brasiliensis* | Third-stage larvae reach lungs about 15 hours after skin penetration. Larvae moult in lungs, pass up respiratory tubes, are swallowed and moult again having reached anterior small intestine. |
| *Oxyspirura mansoni* | Third-stage larvae escape from tissues of intermediate host in crop. Some minutes later, they may be found in the eyes having crawled up oesophagus, across the mouth and along naso-lacrimal ducts. |
| *Spirocerca lupi* | Third-stage larvae penetrate stomach mucosa and, after about 3 weeks, reach wall of aorta via gastric arteries. Three months later, they emerge from aorta as young adults, penetrate oesophageal wall and re-enter oesophageal wall from lumen. |

### 4.3.1. *Host factors influencing emigrations and site selection*

On reaching the alimentary tract, parasitic worms are subjected to many chemical gradients which vary in response to the nature of the diet and the phases of digestive activity. In fact, the location of populations of the tapeworm *Hymenolepis* can be altered by experimental tinkering with the diet. *Moniliformis* performs an anterior emigration of at least 50 cm in the small intestine of rats. This movement may occur in response to a digestive gradient or some basic features of the rat's digestive physiology; evidence for the occurrence of the emigration has been obtained from rats fed on several diets (5.5).

In a discussion of the effects of the host on emigrations and distribution, it is easier to consider morphological features, since the nature of the terrain usually affects the route and logistics of a journey. In a sample of about 400 wild mink infected with the nematode *Dioctophyma renale*, 86% of the mink had from 1 to 8 worms in the right kidney (table 4.6). Presumably the larval *D. renale* usually leave the small intestine by boring through the wall of the duodenum, which passes much closer to the right than to the left kidney. Similarly, the observation that plerocercoids of the tapeworm *Triaenophorus crassus* are more common in the muscles of the right side of the coregonine fish, may be explained by the fact that the stomach of the fish lies against the right body wall.

Hydatid cysts of the tapeworm *Echinococcus granulosus* are generally recovered from the lungs of ruminants and from the livers of non-ruminants (table 4.6). An explanation for this observation may be found in the micro-anatomy of the intestinal walls of the different hosts. In ruminants, the lymphatic vessel of each villus is relatively large and so it can be entered by the relatively large oncosphere, which can then pass to the lungs via the lymphatic system. In non-ruminants the villous lymphatic vessel is small and the oncosphere is more likely to reach the venous vessel and thus arrive in the liver via the portal vessel. Other examples of how the host's morphology may affect emigrations are summarized in table 4.6.

The age, species, sex and physiological and immunological status of the host appear to influence emigrations and site selection. Oncospheres of the tapeworm *Taenia pisiformis* penetrate the wall of the small intestine more anteriorly in young rabbits than in older rabbits, and the young hosts are more susceptible than older hosts to penetration and to the subsequent development of cysticerci in their tissues. Metacercariae of the digenean fluke *Paragonimus westermani* (table 4.1) excyst in the small intestine of various mammals in addition to man. The young flukes eventually reach the lungs of their hosts, but the routes followed and the duration of the emigration in the different species may be different. Some effects of host sex and physiological status on emigrations are illustrated by the emigrations of *Toxocara canis* in dogs. The eggs of *T. canis*, in keeping with those of other ascaridoid species of nematode, hatch in the dog's small intestine, bore through the intestinal wall and in pups emigrate through the tissues to the lungs, from which they reinvade the alimentary tract by way of the bronchi and trachea. In older dogs, the larval *T. canis* follow a somatic route and become trapped in the host's muscles; about 30% more larvae have been recovered from bitches than from male dogs under experimental conditions. When a bitch becomes pregnant, some of the trapped larvae become activated in their somatic sites and they pass the placenta and invade the tissues of the foetus. Thus, pups infected *in utero* may soon begin to disseminate eggs of *T. canis* into the environment†.

Some evidence indicates that the immunological status of a host can affect an emigration and its consequences. Emigrating worms must be exposed to macrophages, phagocytes and other innate and acquired aspects of a host's immune response when they pass through the tissues. Perhaps some of the emigrations (table 4.6) may follow tracts through immunologically privileged territory, but this is not the case during a secondary infection of *Nippostrongylus* in rats or when schistosomula of *Schistosoma* attempt to travel through monkeys which are already harbouring adult worms (Chapter 9).

### 4.3.2. *Parasite behaviour*

The distribution of worms in their hosts (table 4.1), the termination of emigrations once sites have been reached (table 4.6) and the results of experimental studies suggest that site selection may involve the directed behaviour of some species of worm. At the appropriate time in the host–parasite relationship *Nippostrongylus* can be retrieved from its normal site in the jejunum of rats (fig. 4.5) after being surgically transplanted at an earlier time into either the anterior or posterior part of the small intestine. Adults of the hookworm *Ancylostoma caninum* appear to be able to find their normal site in the jejunum of dogs irrespective of their point of surgical introduction into the small intestine. Observations on the tapeworm *Hymenolepis* in experimental infections in rats have shown that worms of a particular age occupy a particular part of the small intestine. When *Hymenolepis* of known age are transplanted into new hosts, the worms can later be retrieved from the predicted region of the small

† Recently, considerable disquiet has been expressed in the UK about the health hazards to young children, in their homes and public playgrounds, as a result of intimate or unsolicited contact with puppies infected with *Toxocara canis*. The eggs of *T. canis* can hatch in the small intestine of the child and the subsequent emigration of the larvae in the child's tissues is undesirable and sometimes dangerous, especially if the eyes and central nervous system are invaded.

intestine. Similar results have been obtained with the acanthocephalan *Moniliformis*. In another study, *H. microstoma* (table 4.1) which had been detached from the walls of the bile ducts of donor mice, were found to invade the bile ducts of recipient mice on transplantation into the lumen of the small intestine. Adult *Spirocerca lupi* (table 4.1) were found to emigrate from the thoracic cavity of a dog to their normal site in the oesophageal wall following transplantation. This observation suggested that an adult worm had retained its site-finding behaviour and the complex activity needed to ensure that its eggs would pass into the alimentary tract and so out of the host. Finally, fluoroscopic techniques have indicated that when adult *Ascaris*, which do not become attached to the host's intestinal wall, move to a different part of the small intestine, the worm moves head first even if the change is in a posterior direction. Administration of a barium meal to a patient deposits radiopaque material in the nematode as well as the host, and although *Ascaris* normally appear to face the direction of gastrointestinal flow, the worms can be observed to bend back upon themselves before moving posteriorly. This direct observation of the living worm in the living host again indicates that a parasite's behaviour contributes much to its distribution in its host.

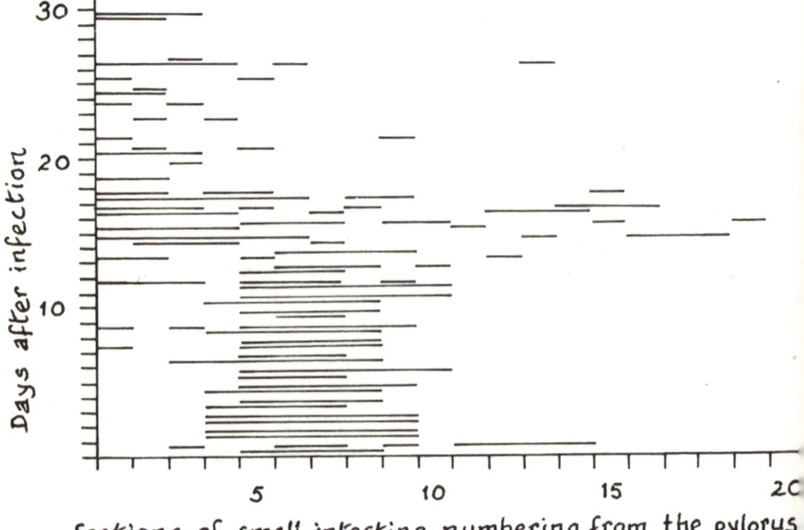


Fig. 4.5. Diagram showing the distribution of *Nippostrongylus brasiliensis* (Nematoda in the small intestines of adequately nourished male and female rats. Observation from female rats are shown by the upper line for each day. The diagram also show how the pattern of distribution changes during the course of a primary infection (afte Brambell, 1965, *Parasitology*, **55**, 313).

# 5. Feeding and nutrition

During the course of evolution, different parasitic worms have become adapted to feed on a wide variety of diets. This specialization, which is a marked feature of parasitism, is reflected in the structure of the parasites' feeding organs and in their feeding activity. In this chapter, most emphasis will be placed on the nature of the diets of adult worms and the methods by which they procure and ingest their food. The feeding activities of worms often damage the host and in certain cases the nutritional demands made by worms on their hosts may also lead to the onset of disease.

## 5.1. *Observations on the diets of worms*

Investigations of the diet and feeding habits of endoparasitic worms in both intermediate and definitive hosts are difficult to conduct because the worms cannot normally be observed *in situ*. Information is usually obtained by four approaches. First, the contents of the alimentary tract of those worms which possess tracts may be examined and compared with the materials present in their sites in the host. Secondly, histological and cytochemical techniques may be applied to worms which have been fixed *in situ* in an attempt to discover how and on what the worms are feeding. Thirdly, a study can be made of the functional morphology of the feeding apparatus and digestive system of a worm in order to determine the likely nature of the diet to which it is adapted. Fourthly, dyes and radioactively labelled substances may be injected into a host with a view to determining the fate of the substances within the parasites. This approach is difficult to use because the marker substances may be metabolized and altered by the host before they reach the parasite. In certain cases, worms may be incubated *in vitro* for short periods with labelled molecules which are suspected of having nutritional significance. Some of the results from these approaches have been summarized in table 5.1.

The smattering of information in table 5.1 supports the idea that the distribution of worms on or in their hosts may be correlated with

TABLE 5.1. *Observations on the food of adult parasitic worms.*

| Parasitic worm | Feeding station | Food |
|---|---|---|
| MONOGENEA | | |
| *Diclidophora merlangi* | Gills of whiting | Blood |
| *Entobdella soleae* | Skin of common sole | Epidermis of skin |
| *Polystoma integerrimum* | Bladder of frog | Blood |
| DIGENEA | | |
| *Apatemon gracilis minor* | Small intestine of duck | Mucus and mucosal tissue |
| *Fasciola hepatica* | Liver and biliary system of sheep | Hepatic and epithelial cells |
| *Haematoloechus medioplexus* | Lungs of frog | Blood |
| *Schistosoma mansoni* | Mesenteric veins of mouse | Blood |
| CESTODA | | |
| *Hymenolepis diminuta* | Small intestine of rat | Digestion products |
| ACANTHOCEPHALA | | |
| *Moniliformis dubius* | Small intestine of rat | Digestion products |
| NEMATODA | | |
| *Ancylostoma caninum* | Small intestine of dog | Blood |
| *Ascaris lumbricoides* | Small intestine of pig | Chyme |
| *Haemonchus contortus* | Abomasum of sheep | Blood |
| *Nippostrongylus brasiliensis* | Small intestine of rat | Mucosal detritus |
| *Tachygonetria stylosa* | Large intestine of tortoise | Bacteria |
| *Trichuris trichiura* | Large intestinal wall of man | Histolysis products |
| *Wuchereria bancrofti* | Lymphatic system of man | Lymph (?) |

the feeding habits of the worms. Cestodes and acanthocephalan worms are nearly always confined to the small intestine of their definitive hosts. Neither type of worm possesses an alimentary tract at any stage of its development, and both must be dependent to a large extent on the host's digestive physiology. Nematodes, however, are able to exploit the wide selection of diets which exist in a vertebrate host (table 5.1) and this degree of feeding specialization is reflected in the structural and functional differences in their alimentary tracts.

Less information is available about the food and feeding habits of the developmental stages of parasitic worms. Many oncomiracidia, miracidia, cercariae and other short-lived stages probably do not feed, but rely for energy on endogenous food reserves. Similarly, metacercariae, third-stage larvae and other long-lived stages, which have completed a phase of development and are essentially inactive, may depend on stored nutrients. Sporocysts and rediae, in contrast, are generative stages and must have high nutritional requirements. Sporocysts (fig. 8.5) probably feed by absorption through their surfaces, whereas rediae (fig. 8.6) possess a mouth and a simple alimentary tract, which has been observed to contain host cells. Many species of nematode experience marked dietary changes during development. For example, the eggs of *Ancylostoma* and *Necator* release free-living larvae which voraciously devour bacteria until they become third-stage larvae. In the host, however, *Ancylostoma* feeds on blood (table 5.1). It is also possible that some of the nematodes which undergo extended emigrations in the tissues of their hosts (table 4.6) may feed on a variety of diets before reaching their permanent sites. Those species which undertake rapid emigrations may not need to feed en route, but they may become more vulnerable to the host's defence reactions if their food reserves reach a critically low level some distance from their destinations.

## 5.2. *Feeding in cestodes and acanthocephalans*

The feeding activities of these two types of worm are considered together since both feed by the absorption of glucose, amino acids and other small molecules which have usually been released by the action of the host's digestive secretions on the host's food or endogenous material. Cestodes and acanthocephalans may also absorb small molecules which have passed from the tissues of the host's mucosa into the intestinal lumen. It is unlikely that these worms ever absorb material directly from the tissues. When oral doses of either radioactively labelled disodium hydrogen phosphate or leucine were given to some rats infected with *Moniliformis* and intraperitoneal doses were given to others, the recovery of radioactivity from the worms was far greater from those in the rats which had swallowed the dose than from those in the injected rats. Experiments of this type indicate that the worms absorb their nutrients from the lumen of the host's intestine.

### 5.2.1. *Feeding apparatus*

Interpretations of the morphology of the body surfaces of cestodes and acanthocephalans have been described in figs. 1.36 and 1.45, and details of the ultrastructure of the absorptive surfaces are shown in figs. 1.33 and 1.46. In both cases, the surface is interpreted as a metabolically active layer bounded by a plasma membrane. The surface of the cestode tegument (fig. 1.33) is composed of very fine processes which are usually called microtriches†. The microtriches resemble the microvilli of the surface of epithelial cells of the vertebrate small intestine (fig. 1.34), whose presence results in an enormous increase in the potential surface area or amount of membrane available for absorption. In rats, the combined effects of having mucosal folding, villi and microvilli have been estimated to increase the surface area of the small intestine by about 600 times. In the tapeworms studied to date, it appears that a ten-fold increase in absorptive surface area is about the maximum effect of the microtriches. The transmission electron microscope often reveals the presence of an electron-dense cone at the end of each microthrix (fig. 1.35). The function of the cones is unknown, but it is possible that their overall effect is to increase friction between the tapeworm and the intestinal wall of the host. In some species, varying sizes of microthrix and varying numbers per unit surface area have been detected from different parts of the strobila.

The surface of an acanthocephalan is very different in appearance from that of a tapeworm (fig. 1.46). The amount of membrane available for absorption has been increased by the development of ramifying membrane-lined channels which are entered through surface pores. Where comparisons have been made, the praesoma appears to possess fewer pores per unit of surface area than the metasoma (fig. 1.39). The acanthocephalan body surface is also coated with a layer of acid mucopolysaccharide, which is probably the material seen in electronmicrographs as a filamentous deposit of about 0.5 μm in thickness (fig. 1.46). Nutrients which pass through the pores cannot be assumed to have been absorbed until they have

† Singular, microthrix.

crossed the membrane lining the channels. Cytochemical studies have also shown that various enzymes are associated with the surface layers of several species of tapeworm and with the acanthocephalan *Moniliformis*. Since cytochemical techniques usually do little more than point to the presence or absence of a substance, quantitative results are often unreliable and information about turnover rates of enzyme activity cannot be obtained. Enzymes may be expected to occur in living tissues and their possible origin and function at the host–parasite interface is discussed below.

### 5.2.2. *Feeding activities*

Our knowledge of how tapeworms and acanthocephalans feed has been obtained from incubating the worms *in vitro* in solutions containing molecules of the type found in the host's small intestine. The change in conditions that a worm will experience when it is transferred from its host's small intestine to an experimenter's flask will be greater than anything Jonathan Swift conjured up for Gulliver. The results, therefore, of studies on the feeding of tapeworms and acanthocephalans indicate the nature of the physiological mechanisms of the worm and not the quantitative importance of the mechanisms, or the identity of preferred food substances.

Tapeworms have been shown *in vitro* to absorb individual amino acids rapidly and against a concentration gradient by an energy-controlled, temperature-dependent process. Kinetic analysis of the experimental results shows that the rate of uptake of a test substance is non-linear with respect to the concentration of the substance in the incubating medium. This finding suggests that some form of carrier molecule or uptake site is involved in the absorption process and that it can become saturated with the substance that is being absorbed. When an uptake mechanism has the features described above, the process is considered to involve active transport. In their natural environment, however, tapeworms are unlikely to be bathed by a solution containing a single amino acid. When the worms are incubated *in vitro* in mixtures of amino acids, it is found that some amino acids competitively inhibit the uptake of others with similar chemical properties, and evidence has been adduced to suggest that several loci or carrier sites exist for the uptake of amino acids in a given tapeworm's surface. Any amino acid might be taken up at any of the loci, but the mutual affinity of a particular amino acid and a particular locus might vary. Consequently, the uptake of amino acids by a tapeworm such as *Hymenolepis*, which possesses at least 4 loci and which may experience different concentrations of 20 amino acids simultaneously, is a complex process which is difficult to investigate.

Much less work has been done on the uptake of amino acids by acanthocephalan worms. By incubating worms *in vitro* with radioactively labelled neutral amino acids, it has been shown that *Moniliformis* actively takes up leucine and probably absorbs it passively as well. *Macracanthorhynchus hirudinaceus* has been found to absorb leucine actively and passively and both *Moniliformis* and *M. hirudinaceus* can take up isoleucine, methionine, alanine and serine *in vitro*. Acanthocephalans have also been reported to absorb glucose, fructose, galactose, mannose, certain disaccharides and glyceryl trioleate amongst other things. The use of autoradiographic methods has indicated that the praesomal surface may not be involved in absorption. An equivalent list could be compiled for tapeworms, although they may not be able to utilize as many types of carbohydrate molecule as acanthocephalan worms. Much work has established, however, that glucose is actively absorbed in an unchanged form *in vitro* by *Hymenolepis*, the rate being affected by the presence or absence of carbon dioxide, the concentration of sodium ions, the hydrogen ion concentration and other factors.

Results from another approach to the study of the feeding mechanisms of tapeworms and acanthocephalan worms have indicated that the relationship between a host's digestive physiology and a worm's mode of feeding may be made more intricate by the activity of enzymes associated with the worm's surface. When *Moniliformis* is incubated *in vitro* with the peptides leucylleucine, leucylglycylglycine, glycylglycine, alanylalanine, tri-alanine and tetra-alanine, amino acids or mixtures of amino acids can be detected in the incubation medium. This hydrolytic activity is related to an aminopeptidase associated with the surface of the worms. Washing them repeatedly with a physiological solution does not reduce the activity, and it appears that the enzyme is a component of the parasite and not an adsorbed secretion of the host. *Moniliformis* also possesses considerable surface amylase activity which can be removed by successive washings and partially restored by immersing the washed worms in luminal contents from the small intestine of rats. Furthermore, the amylytic activity of the enzyme can be inhibited by the presence of rabbit antiserum raised against extracts of rat pancreas. This enzyme, therefore, appears to be a host enzyme which has been adsorbed on to the worm's surface. The properties of acid mucopolysaccharides suggest that the epicuticle of *Moniliformis* (figs. 1.45, 1.46) is well suited for adsorption of enzymes or other molecules. Adsorbed peptides would be located near to surface aminopeptidases and the products of the reaction would probably be released in the vicinity of the worm's amino acid transport system. The possibility of the adsorption of host enzymes onto the tapeworm surface has been raised by the observation that the tapeworms *Hymenolepis diminuta, H. microstoma* and *Moniezia expansa* appear to interact *in vitro* with amylase of endogenous origin. The hydrolysis of starch by amylase seems to be enhanced in some unexplained manner by the presence of the worms. The consequence of such an interaction may be the liberation of small molecules near the absorption sites at the surface of the tapeworms.

Recent studies have also established that tapeworms can take up lipid molecules *in vitro*. *Hymenolepis* can absorb acetate and long-chain saturated and unsaturated fatty acids, and *Spirometra mansonoides* is able to absorb triglyceride molecules as well as fatty acids. Similar results would probably be obtained from most species of cestode and possibly of acanthocephalan. It is interesting to note that the absorption of lipid material *in vitro* by *Hymenolepis* occurs more readily in the presence of bile salts.

### 5.2.3. *Feeding migrations*

In a series of experiments in Texas, the tapeworm *Hymenolepis* was observed to be located in different parts of the rat's small intestine at different times of day. The worms were suspected of changing their positions in response to the feeding routine or digestive activity of the rat. When rats were offered food from 1700 to 0800 hours, the tapeworms occupied the anterior part of the small intestine in the early hours of the morning and the posterior part in late afternoon. Most workers now accept the existence of this regular migration, which may be a component of the tapeworm's feeding activity. We may imagine, for example, that a certain mixture of amino acids may occur in a particular region of the small intestine at a certain time after the host has eaten. We may speculate further that the uptake sites for amino acids at the worm's surface will function most efficiently in the same mixture of amino acids. Clearly, there would be an advantage for the parasite if it could arrive in the region of small intestine when the amino acid concentrations were optimal for feeding. It is not so easy, however, to understand how such a relationship evolved, or to find out the signal which initiates the migration in the small intestine or to explain how the tapeworm receives it. Other worms may also migrate during feeding. The digenean fluke *Podocotyle* sp. is usually found in the anterior part of the small intestine in flounders which have food in their alimentary tracts. The same fluke is found in the rectum of flounders which are kept without food for a few days in an aquarium. Another fluke, *Otodistomum* sp., appears to move between the pyloric and cardiac portions of the stomach of *Raja radiata* in response to the arrival of food in the cardiac portion. The nematode *Contracaecum spiculigerum* has been reported to bury itself deep in the mucosa of the stomach of the black cormorant between meals, and to leave the mucosa and penetrate into the partially digested food which is present soon after the host has fed.

## 5.3. *Feeding in Monogenea and Digenea*

By the time they have reached maturity, many species of monogenean and digenean fluke usually feed either on the blood or on the general epithelial tissues of their hosts (table 5.1). The basic feeding and digestive organs of the two groups of adult fluke are illustrated in figs. 1.4 and 1.8. Food enters through the pharynx, into which may be discharged the contents of various glandular cells. The food then passes into the diverticula of the intestine, which are lined by epithelial cells bearing the characteristic microvilli of an absorptive surface. Histochemical tests have provided some evidence for the activity of phosphatases, esterases and aminopeptidases in the intestinal cells of certain species and it is assumed that these enzymes are somehow involved in the uptake of nutrients from the intestinal lumen, or else in digestion.

### 5.3.1. *Feeding on blood*

The vascular systems of fish, turtles, and birds and mammals are the habitats of the adult forms of certain species of sanguinicolid, spirorchid and schistosomatid fluke, respectively. Not surprisingly these worms swallow and digest blood. Other species of fluke which feed primarily on blood may have to penetrate a blood vessel or damage a vasculated tissue to gain access to their food. A relatively large number of species of monogenean fluke inhabit the gills of fish, and several species of digenean fluke inhabit the lungs of amphibians. In both cases, the flukes are in a region of richly vasculated fragile tissue. The evidence that all these flukes feed on blood is the observation of fresh blood and the digestion products of haemoglobin in the intestines of the living worms. The constituents of the blood plasma are likely to be of equal significance to haemoglobin in the nutrition of the worms concerned.

### 5.3.2. *Feeding on skin derivatives*

Recently, a detailed study has been made of the diet and feeding activity of the monogenean fluke *Entobdella soleae* (table 5.1). Flukes were removed from host fish and fasted for about 24 hours before being returned to the fish. After a brief exploratory period on the surface of the fish, the fluke was observed to grip the host's skin with its haptor. The anterior part of the fluke's feeding apparatus was extruded so as to enclose a small circular area of the host's skin (fig. 5.1). A colourless secretion was then pumped out of the fluke on to the enclosed portion of skin, and after a few minutes this fluid was

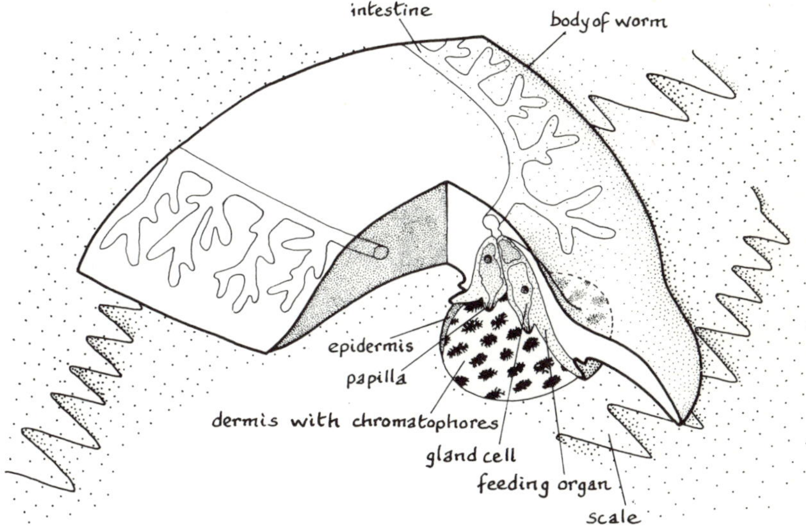


Fig. 5.1. Diagrammatic reconstruction of the anterior region of a specimen of *Entobdella soleae* (Monogenea) in the act of feeding on the skin of its host (after Kearn, 1963, *J. mar. biol. Assn U.K.*, **43**, 749).

sucked into the fluke's intestine and the extrusible portion of the feeding apparatus was withdrawn. This activity removed a small circular portion of epidermis from the host's skin. The dermis was unaffected and undamaged intact chromatophores were visible after feeding had ended. The secretion from the flukes was found to have proteolytic activity, and it would digest the gelatin on a piece of photographic film. Several other species of monogenean fluke appear to feed in the same manner as *E. soleae*. All the flukes which have become specialized for this diet and mode of feeding have unwittingly exploited the fact that the epidermis of a fish regenerates in a few days, so that not only is the food supply replaced but also the fish recovers quickly from the damage caused by the parasites. Both host and parasite would be placed in jeopardy if the parasite were to damage the underlying dermis, which takes about 4 months to recover fully from wounding.

### 5.3.3. *Feeding on tissues and epithelia*

Interpretations of tissue sections from laboratory rodents infected with the common liver-fluke, *Fasciola*, indicate that the young flukes eat their way through the intestinal wall and spend some time feeding on the liver tissues of the host before entering the ducts of the biliary system. Once the young fluke reaches the liver, it appears that the oral sucker grasps a portion of liver tissue, which is pounded to a cellular homogenate by the rapid extrusion and withdrawal of the muscular part of the anterior pharynx. The cellular debris is then sucked into the fluke's intestine. The formation of the homogenate will be enhanced if the fluke secretes histolytic enzymes and if the damaged host tissues release autolytic enzymes. This feeding activity results in the excavation of tunnels which impair the normal functioning of the liver. The initial response of the host is observed to be a massive infiltration of white cells into the region where the flukes are feeding. The presence of the white cells probably increases the damage and contributes still more food for the young flukes. Other evidence suggests that *Fasciola* may be a blood feeder. Blood has been observed in the worm's intestine and experiments with red blood cells which have been labelled with radioactive chromium have indicated that relatively large amounts of blood may be ingested by the flukes. The liver, however, is an extensively vasculated tissue and any organism which eats its way through such tissue is to be expected to ingest blood.

Whereas immature *Fasciola* may spend several weeks in the liver tissues, the adults may spend several years in the biliary system, where their food seems to consist chiefly of the epithelial lining of the ducts. When the flukes enter the liver, changes occur in the bile ducts so that the epithelial cells become enlarged. Thus a lush, cellular pasture develops in preparation for the arrival of the flukes, which now browse on the biliary epithelium for the remainder of their time in association with the host. Again it is possible that flukes will also ingest blood if capillaries in the walls of the bile ducts are pierced. This method of feeding may be typical of other species of fluke which inhabit the livers of mammals.

Other species of digenean fluke browse on epithelial cells but do not seem to cause as much damage to the host as *Fasciola*. Various adult strigeid flukes are characterized by the presence of a cup-shaped forebody which encloses the mouth and attachment organs. *Apatemon gracilis minor* is a strigeid fluke from the small intestine of ducks (table 4.1). During feeding (fig. 5.2), the forebody becomes filled with intestinal mucus as it grips the host's villi. The mucus and enmeshed food particles then enter the fluke's intestine through the mouth in the oral sucker. The villi which are in contact with the attachment organs of the forebody become denuded of epithelial cells and these, or their breakdown products, are no doubt swallowed by the fluke. Histochemical evidence suggests that enzymes released by the fluke are involved in the destruction of the intestinal epithelium. The intestinal epithelium of homoiothermic vertebrates, however, is replaced approximately every 3 days. Thus those worms which feed on intestinal epithelial cells have become adapted to dependence on a food supply in a manner somewhat analogous to that of herbivorous mammals feeding on grass.

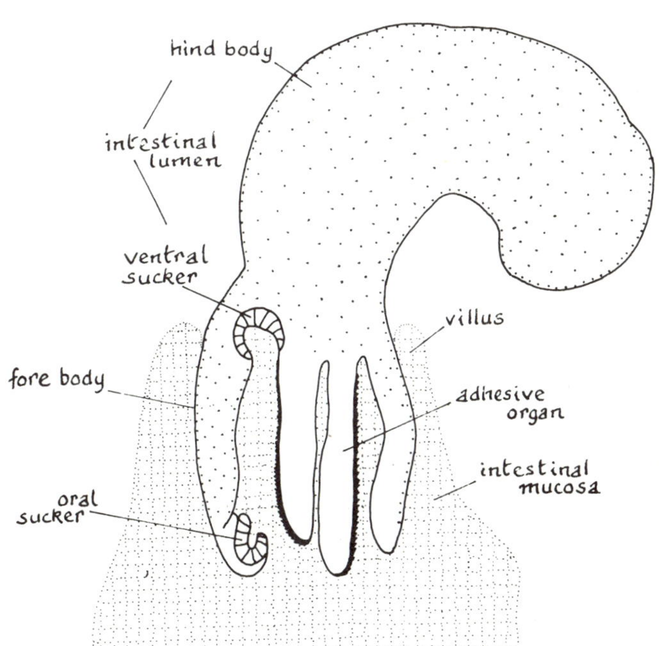


Fig. 5.2. Diagrammatic reconstruction of a specimen of *Apatemon gracilis minor* (Digenea) in the act of feeding on the intestinal mucosa of its host (after Smyth, 1973, *Can. J. Zool.*, **51**, 367).

Examination of flukes with the electron microscope has established that their surface layers must be considered as a tegument of living tissue and not as a toughened cuticle (figs. 1.10, 1.11). Incubation of flukes *in vitro* has demonstrated that materials can be taken up through the tegument. For example, specimens of *Fasciola* with the mouth closed with a ligature can utilize the same amount of glucose *in vitro* as normal flukes. It is, however, extremely difficult to assess the significance of tegumentary absorption in the feeding and nutrition of flukes *in vivo*.

## 5.4. *Feeding in nematodes*

### 5.4.1. *Feeding apparatus*

All known species of nematode possess an alimentary tract which is composed of three main parts. The foregut or stomodaeum includes the mouth, lips, buccal cavity and pharynx. The intestine is a tube lined by a layer of epithelial cells. The hindgut or proctodaeum consists of the rectum and anus in females, and the cloaca with its characteristic copulatory apparatus in male worms. There is little doubt that the alimentary tract is the main route for the entry of nutrients into a nematode's body. Radioactively labelled amino acids fail to enter the body of an *Ascaris* which has had ligatures applied round its mouth and anus, but they are readily detected in the body fluid of unligated worms.

The greatest morphological variation in the nematode alimentary tract is observed in the forebody and in the buccal cavity. Some nematodes possess lips, some stylets, others cutting plates or teeth. This diversity is associated with the varied feeding habits and diets of the worms. The buccal cavity leads into the muscular pharynx and oesophagus, which have a diagnostic appearance for nearly all nematodes when seen in cross section (fig. 1.48). The pharynx functions as a pump which is responsible for the suction of the worm's food into the alimentary system. Many nematodes are too small for convenient study, and detailed work on the functioning of the pharyngeal pump has largely been carried out on *Ascaris* maintained *in vitro* in a special apparatus (figs. 5.3, 5.4). These ingenious gadgets enable worms to be observed and filmed. The pumping capacity of the pharynx can also be determined by measuring the flow of fluid along one capillary tube, through the worm and into the other capillary. It must again be stressed, however, that the behaviour of a worm *in vitro* may be very different from that *in vivo*, and also that the physical properties of a saline solution will be different from those

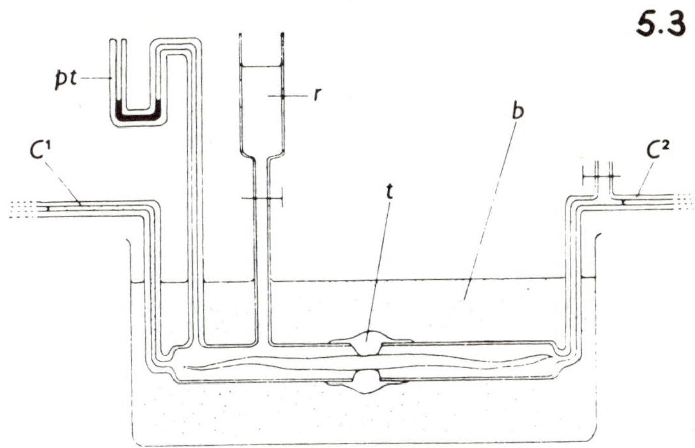


Figs. 5.3 and 5.4. Apparatus for studying the pumping activity of *Ascaris lumbricoides* (Nematoda) *in vitro*. 5.3. Apparatus for measuring the pumping capacity of the pharynx. $C^1$, $C^2$, capillary tubes; b, bath filled with 30% sea water at 38–39 °C; pt, Pitot tube; r, saline reservoir; t, tracheotomy cuff. 5.4 Apparatus for the cinematographic measurement of the uptake of saline from a capillary tube by *Ascaris*. c, capillary tube; l, lens of camera system; pc, perspex cell; s, saline; sc, saline column in the capillary tube; t, tracheotomy cuff; w, worm with anterior end tightly enclosed within the capillary tube (from Mapes, 1966, *Parasitology*, **56**, 137).

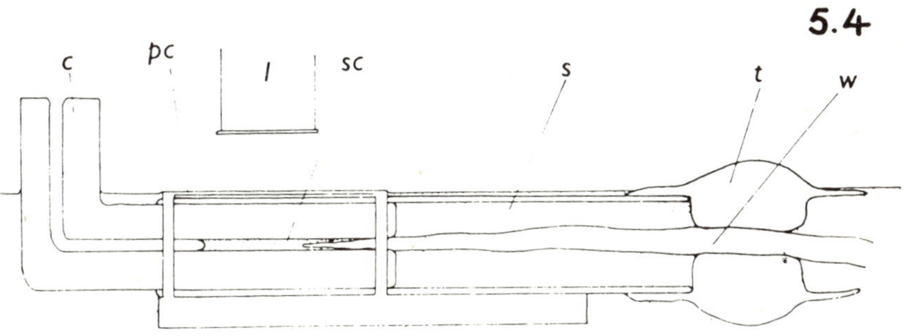


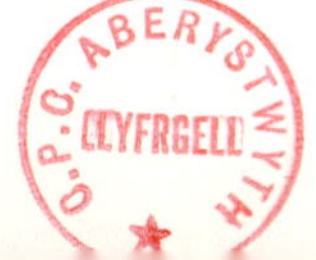

of the intestinal contents which form the normal diet of adult *Ascaris* (table 5.1).

The pumping rate of *Ascaris* is variable. Sometimes the worms pump continuously for several minutes, while at other times bursts of pumping activity are observed with a frequency as high as 20 strokes per second. Typically, the pharynx of *Ascaris* appears to contract about 240 times per minute, and the amount of saline pumped per minute varies from about 38 to 112 $mm^3$. The pumping activity is represented diagrammatically in fig. 5.5. The pharynx of *Ascaris* functions like a simple two-stage pump in which half the pharyngeal lumen is filled with food at any one time. The pattern of the flow of material through the pharynges of other species of nematode is known to be different from that observed when *Ascaris* is ingesting saline. Presumably these differences are related to differences in the type of food ingested. Pumping differences may also occur between developmental stages of the same species if dietary changes occur during development.

An explanation for the functional mechanism of the nematode pharyngeal pump can be deduced from its structure. Contraction of the radial muscles of the pharynx will at first change the triradiate cross-sectional shape of the lumen (fig. 1.48) to that of a triangle. The pharyngeal wall may now 'click' to produce a lumen which is circular in cross section; it is suggested that this 'click' mechanism may be similar in principle to that which is basic to the mechanics of insect flight. In this way, material will be sucked into the worm, with the sequence of pumping (fig. 5.5) being determined by the order in which the pharyngeal muscles contract and relax. The suction force generated by this mechanism is of the order of at least 101 kPa (1 atmosphere). The mean internal pressure of the body fluid within an active *Ascaris* is about 9.3 kPa (70 mmHg), pressures as high as about 50 kPa (half an atmosphere) having been recorded. The force of the pharyngeal pump will easily overcome this internal pressure and propel food past the pharyngeo-intestinal valve into the intestine.

Feeding in *Ascaris* is accompanied by rapid and rather dramatic habits of defaecation. At intervals of 3 or 4 minutes, the anal sphincter of *Ascaris* is relaxed and faecal material may be projected as far as 50 cm. This discharge arises from the combined effects of the powerful pharyngeal pump and the high pressure of the worm's body fluid which is confined within the tough and relatively inextensible cuticle. Although this method of feeding may appear to be wasteful, it should be remembered that in its host the worm probably spends much of its time swimming gently against the flow of chyme. In man, about 10 litres of nutritious fluid pass down the small intestine daily, and if *Ascaris* is present, some of the fluid will be diverted briefly through its intestine, where nutrient molecules will be absorbed. Studies carried out *in vitro* have shown that glucose can be transported from the lumen to the body cavity against a concentration gradient by the intestinal tissues of *Ascaris*.

There is still no consensus of opinion about how material passes along the intestine of parasitic nematodes. In some cases, pharyngeal pumping may force food through the gut, but in others the intestine possesses its own motile properties. The intestine of the mouse pinworm, *Aspiculuris tetraptera*, has been seen to undergo frequent peristaltic-like movements *in vitro*, and ultrastructural evidence has been obtained for the existence of a network of muscle fibres around its intestine.

### 5.4.2. *Feeding activity*

The above account has involved a detailed description of the feeding activity of *Ascaris*, which is probably typical of the species of nematode which feed on the partially digested contents of the host's alimentary tract. Feeding habits associated with blood, tissues and body fluids and bacteria within hosts are equally important.

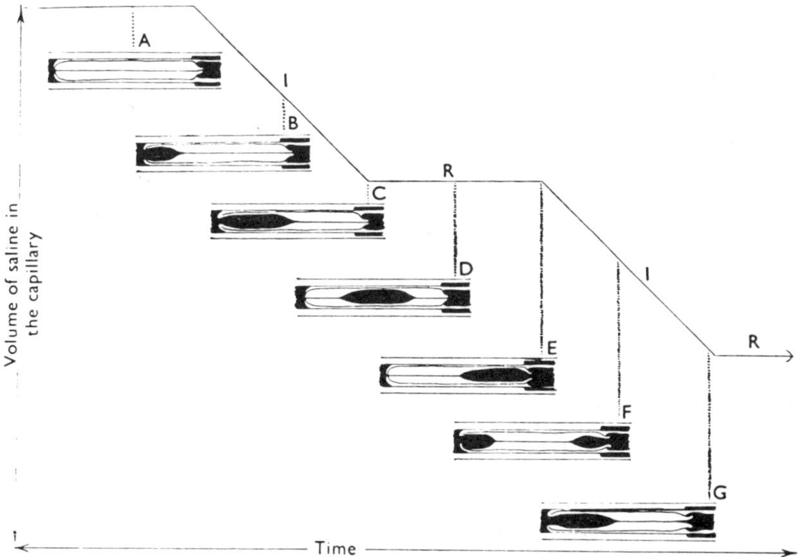


Fig. 5.5. The pumping action of the pharynx of *Ascaris lumbricoides* (Nematoda). I, period of ingestion; R, rest period (no ingestion) (from Mapes, 1966, *Parasitology*, **56**, 137).

5.4.2.1. *Bloodsucking*. Representatives of several genera of nematodes feed on the blood of their hosts or feed in a manner which results in a loss of blood from the host (table 5.1). Most work has been done on hookworms, and there is a correlation between the distribution of hookworm and the occurrence of iron-deficient anaemia in man in tropical countries (Chapter 10). Hookworms grip the intestinal mucosa, lacerate the delicate tissue, and pump the flowing blood into their alimentary tracts. After a time, a worm will release its hold on the mucosa and move to a new feeding site where further haemorrhage is initiated. The discharge of anticoagulants by the worms results in a continuation of bleeding from abandoned feeding sites. Thus the combined effect of haemorrhage from the damaged mucosa and the blood swallowed by the hookworms is to deprive the host of much blood and the iron it contains in association with haemoglobin. One estimate suggests that the global population of hookworms may cause a daily loss of human blood equivalent to about twice the amount used for transfusion purposes each year in the USA.

The dog hookworm, *Ancylostoma caninum*, has been seen to ingest blood *in vivo* in anaesthetized hosts, and blood has been observed in the intestines of hookworms removed from dogs. It is also possible to support a hookworm in a chamber so that its head is surrounded by dog's blood and its anus extends into physiological saline. Blood can be seen to be pumped from one chamber into the other and the amount of blood pumped in this manner can be measured. Furthermore, the worms do not feed *in vitro* unless serum is present in the incubation medium. Many attempts have been made to calculate the amount of blood which is lost by a dog per day as a result of the feeding of *A. caninum*, and quantities varying from 0.015 ml per worm per 24 hours to 0.8 ml per worm per 24 hours have been recorded. This measurement is surprisingly difficult to make, because loss of blood from the host is related to the structure and size of the hookworm population under study (fig. 5.6). Female hookworms remove more blood than males, and an individual worm of either sex tends to remove less in heavy infections than in light infections. Presumably the worms interfere with each others' feeding activity when large numbers are present. The research work which is summarized in part in fig. 5.6 showed that about 1 gram fresh weight of hookworms causes a blood loss of about 65 ml of blood per day from an infected dog. It takes about 500 female or 1200 male *A. caninum* to weigh one gram.

In man, it is generally considered that an individual *Ancylostoma duodenale* causes a greater loss of blood than an individual *Necator americanus*. *Necator*, however, is the more common and more widely distributed hookworm. In domestic ruminants, *Haemonchus contortus* and its relatives feed by blood-letting, and so cause distress to both their hosts and the farmers.

5.4.2.2. *Feeding on tissues and body fluids*. Whipworms of the genus *Trichuris* (fig. 1.55, table 5.1) burrow into the wall of the large intestine of the host and it appears that they secrete substances which dissolve the host's tissues and so produce a nutrient soup which is pumped into the worm. Small blood vessels are also likely to be damaged by this feeding process and blood may also be ingested by the worm or lost by the host. *Trichinella spiralis* is a small nematode with a buccal stylet which would appear to be used for piercing lymphatic or blood vessels in the mucosa so that a nutrient fluid is released for the worms to ingest. Many years ago a study of *T. spiralis* in hamsters revealed that protozoa of the genus *Giardia* have a

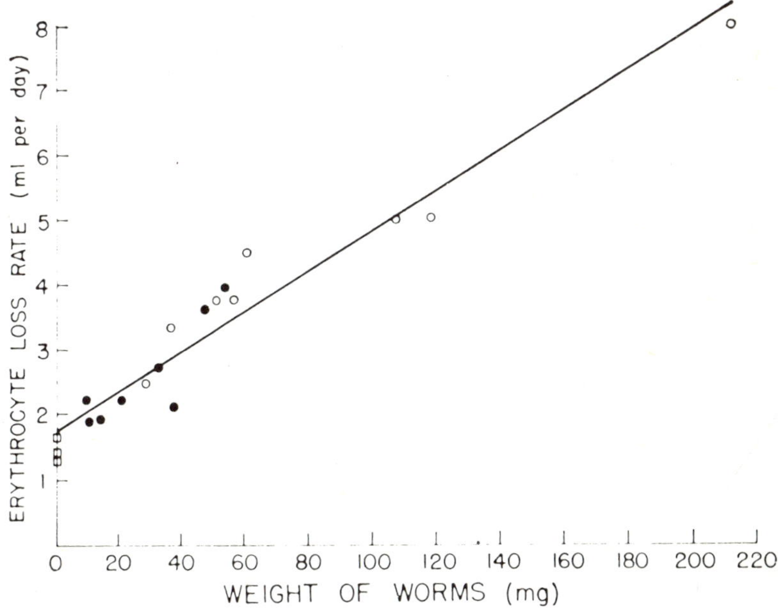


Fig. 5.6. Erythrocyte loss rate from dogs (ml per day) as a function of the total weight of individual burdens of *Ancylostoma caninum* (Nematoda). Open circles represent female worms; closed circles represent male worms; squares represent control (uninfected) values (from Georgi, LeJambre and Ratcliffe, 1969, *J. Parasit.*, **55**, 1205).

tendency to congregate around the anal openings of the feeding nematodes. Perhaps the protozoa utilize the nutrients which pass from the host through the worm. Presumably adult filarial nematodes like *Wuchereria bancrofti* ingest the body fluids in which they are bathed (table 5.1).

5.4.2.3. *Feeding on bacteria*. Several species of nematode which reach adulthood in the large intestine of vertebrates probably continue to depend on the microbivorous habit which characterized their period of free-living development. The vertebrate large intestine contains vast numbers and types of micro-organisms, and it is usual to find at least $10^9$ cells per gram fresh weight of intestinal contents. These cells probably form an important item in the diet of *Heterakis, Enterobius, Aspiculuris, Syphacia* and many more genera. Some species of nematode may be able to co-exist in the large intestine because they have become specialized to one of the many potential diets which are to be found there. *Tachygonetria stylosa* and *T. robusta* share the same site in the colon of the tortoise (fig. 4.3), but *T. stylosa* eats bacteria whereas *T. robusta* feeds indiscriminately on intestinal contents.

## 5.5. *Nutritional requirements of worms*

In contrast to many micro-organisms, which have the ability to synthesize complex molecules from simple ones, most animals require at least 40 chemical compounds or inorganic elements if their metabolic demands for energy and for growth, repair, reproduction and general physiology are to be met. The amount of each nutrient which is required may vary according to the developmental stage of the organism and the chemical composition of the diet. A growing chicken needs to eat a diet containing about 210 g protein per kg provided that about 12 000 kJ (2 800 kcal) of metabolizable energy are available from each kg of diet. On the other hand, 1 kg of the same diet should contain about 50 mg of zinc and as little as 0.05 parts per million of selenium, provided that the concentration of certain other nutrients remains at a satisfactory level. At present, we have very superficial and incomplete knowledge of the nutritional requirements of parasitic worms. Those worms which feed on bacteria, tissues or body fluids are very likely to receive an adequate diet for the propagation and maintenance of their species irrespective of their stage of development or the state of the host. Even when hosts are undernourished and suffering from extreme stress, parasites seem to flourish, and plague, pestilence and famine have been related ever since man recorded his history. Any worm which ingests and digests host tissues is likely to obtain carbohydrates, lipids, proteins, vitamins, inorganic substances and water. Unfortunately, the nutritional requirements of the worms are unlikely to be determined until they can be grown *in vitro*, in chemically defined media which do not contain yeast or liver extracts or various types of sera. Paradoxically, the achievement of growing a worm *in vitro* in a defined medium would automatically solve the problem of establishing the nutritional requirements of the worm in question.

Some information is available, however, about the nutrition of tapeworms and acanthocephalans in their definitive hosts. These worms are directly dependent on the hydrolysis of the host's diet and they are likely, therefore, to be sensitive to its experimental modification. Depriving the host of protein in the short term has no obvious effect. The worms are assumed to meet their requirements from the endogenous sources of nitrogen which are released into the small intestine. Tapeworms usually contain high levels of reserve polysaccharide (table 6.2), and it was discovered over 30 years ago that the polysaccharide content of *Raillietina cesticillus* in domestic fowl fell to about 11% of the normal value when the birds were fasted for a short time, while proglottides of the tapeworm were shed. Similar observations were made on *Hymenolepis*. When rats infected with this worm are maintained on a carbohydrate-deficient diet for 2 weeks, many of the worms pass out of the hosts and the survivors cease to produce eggs and weigh very much less than those which have continued to thrive in similar rats feeding on an adequate diet. Under experimental conditions, involving carefully chosen numbers of *Hymenolepis*, the size and reproductive rate of this tapeworm appear to be directly related to the dietary carbohydrate intake of the rat. The quality and quantity of the carbohydrate ingested by the host also affect *Hymenolepis*. Starch is better for the tapeworm than the equivalent quantity of either glucose or sucrose in the rat's diet. Presumably more glucose is likely to be available to the worm from the starch which must be digested, than when glucose itself is ingested by the host. The absorption of glucose may occur in the anterior part of the host's tract where *Hymenolepis* is not to be found. Similarly, the hydrolysis of sucrose to glucose and fructose will occur more rapidly than that of starch, and it seems that *Hymenolepis* may not utilize fructose *in vitro*. The intake of dietary starch by the rat is not the only requirement for the welfare of *Hymenolepis*. It is important, for example, that adequate roughage or fibre should be included in the diet; this finding suggests that the physicochemical conditions prevailing in the tract during digestion must be very important to the parasites.

Other species of intestinal worm are also sensitive to the dietary carbohydrate intake of their hosts. *Hymenolepis nana* from mice and *H. citelli* from hamsters do not grow if carbohydrate is omitted from the host's diet, and the nematode *Ascaridia galli* seems to be more vigorous when living in fowls which are ingesting carbohydrate.

Many of the points mentioned above can be illustrated by reference to a detailed study of the relationship between the growth of the acanthocephalan *Moniliformis* and the carbohydrate intake of rats. Four isoenergetic diets (table 5.2) were designed and a population of male rats of the same pedigree was acclimatized to each of the diets. The rats were then infected with the same strain of *Moniliformis* and the state of the host–parasite relationship with regard to the four diets compared by examining the infected rats at weekly intervals from 1 to 18 weeks post infection. A selection of the results is summarized in table 5.3. It can be seen that the rat's diet did not affect the activation of the cystacanths of *Moniliformis* nor the establishment of the worms in the posterior part of the small intestine. The anteriorly directed emigration of the worms in the small intestine (table 4.6) also occurred irrespective of the diet, but subsequently differences were observed in the distribution of the worms in the small intestines of the rats fed on diets C and D (table 5.3). After 4 weeks, consistently fewer *Moniliformis* were recovered from the rats fed on diets A and B than from the rats fed on diets C and D. Differences were also noted in the longevity of the surviving worms in the rats fed on the different diets (table 5.3). Perhaps the most striking differences were observed in the growth and reproduction of the worms. *Moniliformis* from rats

TABLE 5.2. *Composition of four isoenergetic diets used in a study of the nutrition of* Moniliformis *(Acanthocephala) in the small intestine of rats (after Nesheim, Crompton, Arnold and Barnard, 1977).*

| | Ingredients of diets (g kg$^{-1}$) | | | |
|---|---|---|---|---|
| | A | B | C | D |
| Maize starch | — | — | 36 | 586.5 |
| Powdered cellulose | 314.5 | 323.5 | 294.5 | — |
| Maize oil | — | 383 | — | 120 |
| Fatty acids from maize oil | 392 | — | 376 | — |
| Protein (casein) | 232 | 232 | 232 | 232 |
| Vitamins, minerals, etc. | 61.5 | 61.5 | 61.5 | 61.5 |

TABLE 5.3. *Observations on the course of infection of* Moniliformis *(Acanthocephala) in rats fed on isoenergetic diets (table 5.2) (after Nesheim, Crompton, Arnold and Barnard, 1977).*

| | Time (weeks) | Host diet A | B | C | D |
|---|---|---|---|---|---|
| Mean number of worms in a rat. Each rat was given a dose of 20 cystacanths. | 1 | 12.5 | 14.25 | 14.25 | 14.75 |
| | 4 | 11.5 | 15.25 | 13.0 | 16.75 |
| | 8 | 6.75 | 3.25 | 12.25 | 9.0 |
| | 11 | 0.25 | 0 | 1.75 | 1.75 |
| | 16 | 0 | 0 | 3.25 | 1.0 |
| Mean attachment position of the worms in the rats. The numbers represent the percentage of the distance along the small intestine from the stomach. 50 is half way. | 1 | 80 | 70 | 68 | 68 |
| | 4 | 24 | 35 | 28 | 32 |
| | 8 | 29 | 27 | 22 | 59 |
| | 11 | 14 | — | 33 | 45 |
| | 16 | — | — | 29 | 49 |
| Mean dry weights (mg) of female worms. Values with an asterisk show the sex could not be determined by direct inspection. | 1 | 0.1* | 0.1* | 0.1* | 0.1* |
| | 4 | 1.0* | 0.8* | 5.3 | 9.5 |
| | 8 | 4.0 | 3.5 | 36.3 | 34.9 |
| | 11 | 12.0 | — | 47.5 | 30.5 |
| | 16 | — | — | 93.6 | 61.0 |

fed on diets A and B hardly grew at all and it was very difficult to decide which were males and which were females. The gonads of such worms did not develop and no eggs were found. Worms from rats fed on diet D grew more rapidly than those from the rats fed on diet C, but gradually the *Moniliformis* from the rats fed on diet C grew bigger and presumably produced eggs for a longer time (table 5.3). In rats fed on diet C or on diet D, reproduction and egg release by the worms were normal. It must be emphasized that the growth and health of the rats, which were assessed by measuring weight gain, food-intake and size of the small intestine, were satisfactory and very similar.

Other species of worm, for example *Schistosoma* spp., are dependent on glucose, but the fact that they inhabit the blood of their hosts means that any attempt to experiment with their glucose requirements *in vivo* might place the host in danger long before the parasite was affected. Further aspects of the importance of carbohydrates to parasitic worms are considered in the next chapter.

# 6. Energy metabolism

Animals obtain most of their energy for chemical and physical work by the oxidation of relatively stable and complex molecules, which may have been stored in the body or may have been provided directly from the diet. This process of oxidation is achieved through a sequence of enzymic reactions leading to the synthesis of adenosine triphosphate (ATP), which is the main energy currency of the cell.

Biological oxidation can conveniently be considered as the loss of hydrogen rather than the gain of oxygen. Similarly, reduction is the gain of electrons rather than the loss of oxygen.

## 6.1. *Energy metabolism of free-living animals*

The significance of the energy metabolism of parasitic worms is difficult to appreciate without a discussion of the salient features of energy metabolism in free-living animals. Many of these are dependent on oxygen, which acts as the electron acceptor in the final stages of energy metabolism. Thus, foodstuffs are broken down to energy, carbon dioxide and water. A simplified scheme for the breakdown of glucose in the cell is shown in figs. 6.1 and 6.2. The evidence for this concept is extremely strong, and has been obtained from studies *in vivo* and *in vitro* involving the detection and extraction of intermediate compounds and enzymes, the use of enzyme inhibitors, the introduction of radioactively labelled metabolites, and the application of the human genius.

The first phase of energy metabolism consists of the breakdown of glucose to pyruvate (fig. 6.1). This process, which is known as glycolysis, occurs in the cytoplasm, where enzymic activity is required during the conversion of one metabolite to the next. Some of the enzymes, for example glyceraldehyde 3-phosphate dehydrogenase, which catalyses the conversion of glyceraldehyde 3-phosphate to 1,3-diphosphoglycerate, do not function without the participation of a cofactor. In this case, the cofactor is nicotinamide adenine dinucleotide ($NAD^+$) which accepts electrons and a proton from the

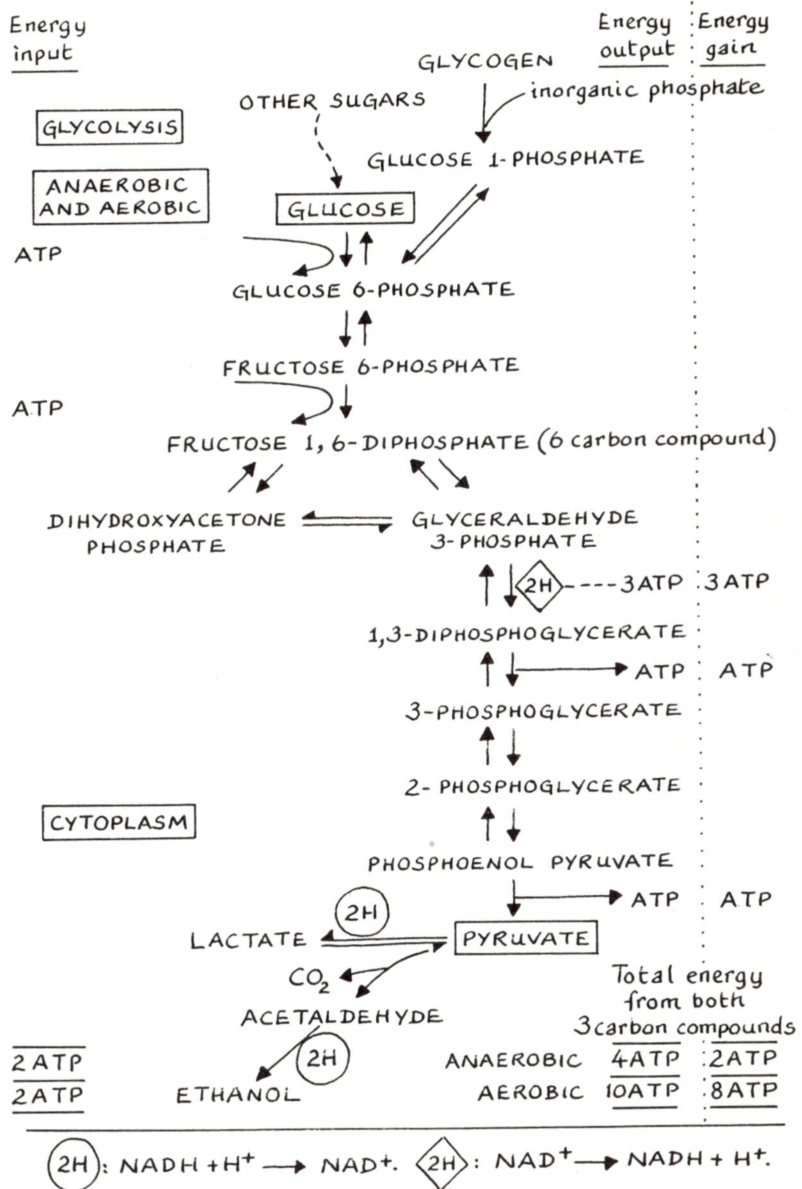


Fig. 6.1. A flow diagram showing the main steps in glycolysis which is the breakdown of glucose to pyruvate.

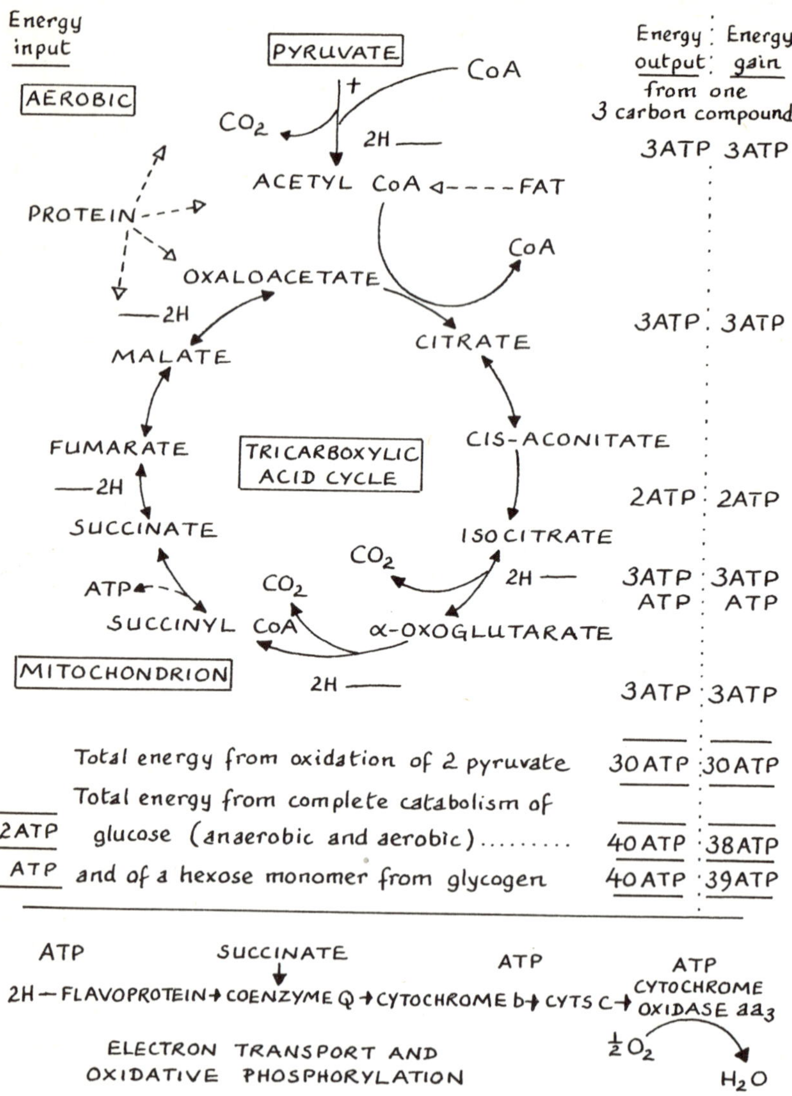


† IN SOME ANAEROBIC ORGANISMS, PYRUVATE MAY GO TO EITHER ACETYL CoA OR ACETYL PHOSPHATE, BOTH HIGH ENERGY COMPOUNDS, USING FERREDOXIN AS THE ELECTRON ACCEPTOR AND PRODUCING HYDROGEN.

Fig. 6.2. A flow diagram showing the main steps in the tricarboxylic acid cycle. Details of electron transport and oxidative phosphorylation are also shown.

aldehyde group of the glyceraldehyde 3-phosphate. The reduced form of nicotinamide adenine dinucleotide ($NADH + H^+$) is an extremely important compound in the transfer of electrons, which is after all the essence of biological oxidation–reduction.

The glycolytic pathway functions in the absence of oxygen as long as pyruvate is removed and the reduced cofactors are regenerated. In mammals, pyruvate can be converted to lactate, with the regeneration of $NAD^+$ (fig. 6.1) and this mechanism is important during periods of intense muscular activity, when cells use their oxygen faster than it can be replaced. Soon after the activity has subsided, oxygen consumption increases above the normal rate until the oxygen debt has been repaid. What happens is that some of the accumulated lactate is cleared by converting it back to pyruvate, which is then metabolized through the tricarboxylic acid cycle whose functioning is indirectly linked to a supply of oxygen. In yeast, the pyruvate is removed by converting it to ethanol (fig. 6.1), and $NAD^+$ is again regenerated and made available for use elsewhere in the glycolytic pathway or in other reactions in the cell.

The next series of reactions in energy metabolism concern the tricarboxylic acid cycle (fig. 6.2). Pyruvate combines with coenzyme A (CoA) through the action of the enzymes of the pyruvate dehydrogenase system to form acetyl coenzyme A. This compound combines with oxaloacetate to form citrate, which contains six carbon atoms. As the reactions proceed, two carbon atoms are lost in the form of carbon dioxide, oxaloacetate being reformed to combine with more acetyl coenzyme A. In this way, carbon in gradually removed from the glucose which gave rise to the pyruvate. The breakdown of the intermediate compounds of the tricarboxylic acid cycle releases pairs of hydrogen atoms at four places in the cycle (fig. 6.2). The importance of the tricarboxylic acid cycle in the energy metabolism of aerobic cells is that the pair of hydrogen atoms are passed by reduced cofactors to the electron transport or transfer system of the mitochondrion where most ATP is produced. The hydrogen is passed from the reduced cofactors, by means of coenzyme Q and the cytochrome enzymes, to oxygen which functions as the final electron acceptor with the formation of water (fig. 6.2). During the passage of the electrons from hydrogen to oxygen the energy which is released is trapped by the formation of ATP; this process is known as oxidative phosphorylation. Electron transport and oxidative phosphorylation occur in association with the membranes or cristae of the mitochondrion.

It can be calculated from the information in fig. 6.1 that the breakdown of free glucose to pyruvate by glycolysis anaerobically provides the cell with a net gain of two molecules of ATP for every molecule of glucose, while the breakdown of glucose originating from glycogen provides three molecules of ATP. Once oxygen is available, however, and electron transport and oxidative phosphorylation can function in conjunction with the tricarboxylic acid cycle, many more molecules of ATP can be synthesized in addition to those produced during glycolysis. In terms of the strategy of metabolic evolution, any cell living under conditions of near anaerobiosis would appear to require an abundant supply of glucose, mechanisms for regenerating reduced cofactors and some method of excreting the end-products of glucose degradation. The cell which is equipped to live in the aerobic situation will require less glucose, particularly since fats and, under certain conditions, proteins can also be degraded for energy, provided that oxygen is ultimately available as the electron acceptor (fig. 6.2).

## 6.2 *Energy metabolism of adult worms*

### 6.2.1. *Experimental methods*

One approach to studying the energy metabolism of parasitic worms is to incubate them with radioactively labelled glucose in a sealed vessel under known conditions. After a given time, the vessel is opened, the fate of the labelled substrate is determined, and hypotheses are suggested to explain how the metabolites could have acquired the radioactive label. This technique is valuable because it enables reproducible results to be obtained by the investigator and by other workers, but the procedure and interpretation of the results are restricted by a major drawback. At present, it is impossible to simulate *in vitro* the conditions which exist in a worm's living microhabitat. For example, although oxygen is intimately involved in energy metabolism (fig. 6.2), it is difficult to know how much is available to the worms. Some live in the vertebrate bloodstream and tissues (table 4.1), where oxygen is usually available, and some live in or near the intestinal mucosa, where they will be exposed to the oxygen which diffuses out of the intestinal cells. Other species of worm, in contrast, live in the intestinal contents of the large intestine, where there may be no detectable oxygen. Difficulties arise in making reliable measurements of the oxygen tension in a worm's microhabitat, and even greater difficulties would be encountered if attempts were made to subject the worms *in vitro* to a constant oxygen tension like that prevailing *in vivo*.

Despite technical limitations, much information has been obtained about the metabolic processes of worms *in vitro*. An example that shows how the biochemistry of worms may be studied is given by a recent investigation of *H. contortus*, the adults of which live swathed in mucus in close association with the wall of the sheep's abomasum, from which they ingest blood. They are therefore exposed to oxygen and the other substances which may diffuse out of the abomasal wall, and to the physicochemical conditions in the abomasal lumen. In addition, their diet gives them a steady supply of glucose at a concentration in the blood of about 60 mg per 100 ml of blood together with oxygen bound to haemoglobin and in solution in the blood plasma. In one experiment, the investigator confined a number of fresh, 85-day-old *Haemonchus*, weighing 0.63 g, for 5 hours in a balanced salt solution containing radioactively labelled glucose† in the apparatus shown in fig. 6.3. Care was taken to adjust the pH, temperature and osmotic pressure of the medium to values similar to those occurring during the host–parasite relationship. The initial oxygen tension in the incubation medium was 2.5 kPa (19 mmHg), but it was found, by means of an oxygen electrode, that no oxygen could be detected in the medium 20 minutes after the beginning of the experiment. The

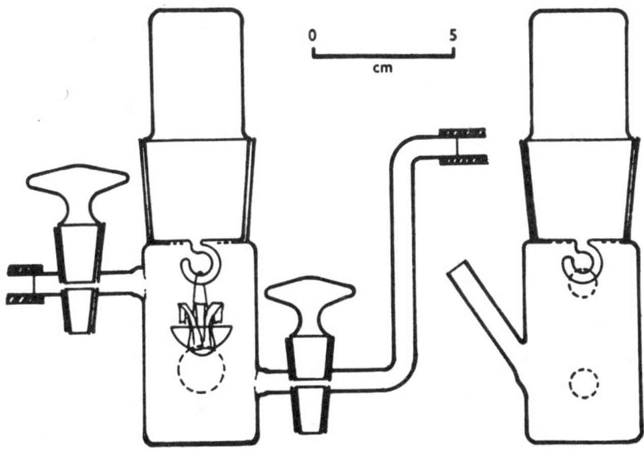


Fig. 6.3. Apparatus for the *in vitro* incubation of adult *Haemonchus contortus* (Nematoda) with D-[U-$^{14}$C] glucose. Two views are shown, one at right angles to the other. The broken-lined rings shown on one view indicate the position of the side arms shown on the other view. The two stop-cocked side-arms were used initially for gassing the apparatus and the third side-arm for mounting a small oxygen electrode using a gas-tight neoprene O-ring. The alkali trap (for $CO_2$ absorption) was suspended from a hook on the stopper (from Ward, 1974, *Parasitology*, **69**, 175).

† D-[U-$^{14}$C]Glucose, in which U-$^{14}$C denotes statistically uniform labelling of each carbon atom in the glucose molecule with the radioisotope $^{14}$C.

worms were assumed to have used the oxygen, and the remaining experimental period of 4 hours 40 minutes was conducted under conditions of near anaerobiosis. The fate of the radioactive glucose during the experiment is shown in table 6.1. Overall, 98.8% of the original quantity of radioactivity was accounted for, and glucose was shown to have been converted to carbon dioxide and a variety of complex end-products, the nature and significance of which are discussed below.

TABLE 6.1. *Recovery of radioactivity (μCi) from an incubation of adult* Haemonchus contortus *(Nematoda) with* D-*[U-*$^{14}$*C]glucose* in vitro *(after Ward, 1974).*

| | |
|---|---|
| Radioactivity in medium at start | 25.25 |
| Radioactivity in medium at end[a] | 17.36 |
| Radioactivity in worm washings[a] | 5.39 |
| Radioactivity condensed in vessel (fig. 6.3) | 0.01 |
| Radioactivity in $CO_2$ trap (fig. 6.3) | 0.002 |
| Radioactivity in expired $CO_2$ | 0.74 |
| Radioactivity inside worms | 1.44 |
| Total | 24.942 |
| Percentage recovery of radioactivity | 98.8 |

[a] In addition to $CO_2$, radioactive end-products of glucose metabolism were identified at the end of the experiment as follows: propanol 0.69, ethanol 0.07, propionate 1.00, acetate 0.53, succinate 0.07 and lactate 0.04 μCi.

### 6.2.2. *General aspects of glucose metabolism*

Circumstantial and direct evidence indicates that the glycolytic breakdown of carbohydrate to pyruvate (fig. 6.1) is the basis of energy metabolism in many parasitic worms. Several worms have a nutritional requirement for carbohydrate (5.5). Some species contain large amounts of stored carbohydrate (table 6.2) and, after periods of starvation, high priority is given to its replenishment. For example, in starved specimens of *Hymenolepis*, 40% of the glucose consumed during the first 15 minutes of its reintroduction into the experimental system is converted to glycogen. The activity of worms *in vitro* under anaerobiosis is often enhanced and prolonged by the inclusion of glucose in the incubation medium. The end-products of glucose metabolism *in vitro* may or may not include carbon dioxide, but incomplete oxidation products are produced (table 6.3), irrespective of the presence or absence of oxygen in the experimental conditions. In the experiment with *Haemonchus contortus* (described above), the

TABLE 6.2. *Estimations of the polysaccharide (glycogen) content of some adult parasitic worms (after von Brand, 1973).*

| Parasitic worm | Site and host (table 4.1) | Polysaccharide[a] (% dry weight) |
|---|---|---|
| MONOGENEA | | |
| *Diclidophora merlangi* | Gills of fish | 1.2 |
| *Polystoma integerrimum* | Bladder of frog | 8.5 |
| DIGENEA | | |
| *Fasciola hepatica* | Biliary system of sheep | 15–21 |
| *Schistosoma mansoni* male | Mesenteric vessels of mouse | 14–29 |
| *Schistosoma mansoni* female | Mesenteric vessels of mouse | 3–5 |
| CESTODA | | |
| *Hymenolepis diminuta* | Small intestine of rat | 26–48 |
| *Moniezia expansa* | Small intestine of sheep | 24–32 |
| ACANTHOCEPHALA | | |
| *Moniliformis dubius* | Small intestine of rat | 2.3–24 |
| NEMATODA | | |
| *Ascaris lumbricoides* | Small intestine of pig | 14–24 |
| *Litomosoides carinii* | Pleural cavity of cotton rat | 5 |
| *Nippostrongylus brasiliensis* | Small intestine of rat | 3.3 |

[a] These measurements may vary according to the diet and nutritional status of the host.

radioactive end-products were identified as propanol, ethanol, propionate, acetate, succinate and lactate. Excretion of substances such as these suggests that the energy production of the worms is not always dependent on the complete terminal pathways which have been detected in free-living organisms (fig. 6.2). Furthermore, excretion of metabolites such as lactate means that an oxygen debt does not develop. *Schistosoma mansoni* lives in the venous blood of its host, but under *in vitro* conditions all the glucose that it metabolizes can be accounted for as lactate (table 6.3), which has been formed by glycolysis even though oxygen is present. Other worms, for example the tapeworm *Taenia taeniaeformis* from the small intestine of the cat, appear to metabolize less carbohydrate *in vitro* when oxygen is available (table 6.4). Finally, most of the enzymes known to be involved in glycolysis have been shown to be active in homogenates prepared from the tissues of worms, including *Fasciola, Schistosoma, Hymenolepis* and *Ascaris*.

There is much interest in whether the adult stages of various species of parasitic worm have a functional tricarboxylic acid (TCA) cycle (fig. 6.2). Seven of the enzymes of the TCA cycle have been detected

TABLE 6.3. *End-products of the energy metabolism of adult endoparasitic worms* in vitro *(after von Brand, 1973).*

| Parasitic worm | Anaerobic or at very low oxygen tension | | | | | | | | | | With oxygen | | | | | | | | | |
|---|---|---|---|---|---|---|---|---|---|---|---|---|---|---|---|---|---|---|---|---|
| | Acetate | Formate | Lactate | Propionate | Pyruvate | Succinate | $C_4$ acids | $C_5$ acids | $C_6$ acids | Ethanol | Acetate | Formate | Lactate | Propionate | Pyruvate | Succinate | $C_4$ acids | $C_5$ acids | $C_6$ acids | Ethanol |
| DIGENEA | | | | | | | | | | | | | | | | | | | | |
| *Fasciola hepatica* | + | | (+) | + | | | (+) | (+) | | | + | | (+) | + | | + | (+) | (+) | | |
| *Schistosoma mansoni* | | | + | | | | | | | | | | + | | | | | | | |
| CESTODA | | | | | | | | | | | | | | | | | | | | |
| *Hymenolepis diminuta* | + | | + | | | + | | | | | | | + | | | | | | | |
| *Moniezia expansa* | | | + | | | + | | | | | | | + | | | + | | | | |
| *Taenia taeniaeformis* | + | | + | | (+) | + | | | | + | + | | + | | + | + | | | | (+) |
| ACANTHOCEPHALA | | | | | | | | | | | | | | | | | | | | |
| *Moniliformis dubius* | + | (+) | + | (+) | | + | + | | | + | + | + | + | | | + | | | | + |
| NEMATODA | | | | | | | | | | | | | | | | | | | | |
| *Ascaris lumbricoides* | | (+) | (+) | | | + | + | + | + | | + | (+) | (+) | + | | + | + | + | | |

\+ Present in a significant amount
(+) Present in a very small amount

TABLE 6.4. *Observations on the carbohydrate metabolism of adult* Taenia taeniaeformis *(Cestoda)* in vitro *(after von Brand, 1973).*

| | |
|---|---|
| Glucose consumption (exogenous carbohydrate) | |
| Aerobic | 0.07 μmole/mg dry tissue/h |
| Anaerobic | 0.10 μmole/mg dry tissue/h |
| Glycogen consumption (endogenous carbohydrate) | |
| Aerobic | 6.48 g/100 g wet weight of tapeworm/24 h |
| Anaerobic | 9.36 g/100 g wet weight of tapeworm/24 h |

in the tissues of adult *Fasciola*, and citrate, aconitate, α-oxoglutarate, succinate, fumarate, malate and oxaloacetate have also been found in homogenates of the fluke's tissue. It is difficult to estimate how important this pathway may be in the energy metabolism of the adult flukes in the bile ducts of their hosts. The role of the cycle in energy production depends ultimately on oxygen as the acceptor of electrons from the reduced cofactors. *Fasciola* and some of the worms mentioned above and in the tables are relatively large and thus their ratios of surface area to volume may not favour gaseous exchange. Parasitic worms also lack a pumped circulatory system and no clear respiratory function has been demonstrated for the haemoglobin which is found in *Ascaris* and other worms. At present, therefore, it is difficult to decide whether the complete TCA cycle contributes significantly to the energy metabolism of all adult endoparasitic worms *in vivo*.

This conclusion may be difficult to reconcile with the fact that many worms consume oxygen when it is available, and that the oxygen does not always seem to suppress glycolysis (table 6.3). In some cases, however, the oxygen does have an effect on metabolism, although the biochemical pathways are not fully understood. Adults of the filarial nematode *Litomosoides carinii* live in the oxygenated pleural cavity of cotton rats (table 4.1). *In vitro*, oxygen is needed for its motility and survival and it consumes oxygen at an increased rate if it has previously been kept under nitrogen. *Nippostrongylus*, which is a small nematode with a large surface area relative to its volume, lives in contact with the mucosa of the rat's small intestine. Lactate is the major end-product of its endogenous carbohydrate metabolism, but the quantities produced differ according to the presence or absence of oxygen in the incubation system. More carbohydrate is used and more lactate is formed in a given time when air is absent than when it is present.

The adult stages of *H. contortus* and other species of parasitic worm either require oxygen or consume it when it is available. Worms like *Haemonchus* are curious in that they possess mitochondria of different appearance (figs. 6.4, 6.5). Mitochondria with many cristae (fig. 6.5) are usually found in tissues where aerobic processes (fig. 6.2) occur, whereas mitochondria with few cristae (fig. 6.4) are sometimes assumed to indicate that oxidative phosphorylation is insignificant in the tissues concerned. As can be seen from figs. 6.6. and 6.7, mitochondria from equivalent tissues in different worms can be very different in appearance. Furthermore, functional cytochromes have been detected and the existence of oxidative phosphorylation has been demonstrated with preparations of mitochondria from the large tapeworm *Moniezia expansa*. This miscellany of observations sugests that adult parasitic worms have a wide range of biochemical options available, and that they may be best considered as metabolic opportunists.

The evolution of reactions which lead to the formation and excretion of molecules such as succinate (table 6.3) illustrates this concept of metabolic opportunism. Succinate production has been investigated in detail in the muscles of *Ascaris*, whose main pathways of carbohydrate catabolism are summarized in fig. 6.8. The important features are that carbon dioxide is fixed to form oxaloacetate which is converted to malate with the regeneration of cofactor. The malate is further metabolized in the mitochondrion to provide succinate which is formed in conjunction with ATP. Thus there is a mechanism for the regeneration of cofactor and for the production of ATP without the participation of oxygen. The fumarate reductase involved in this reaction (fig. 6.8) should not be confused with succinate dehydrogenase which catalyses the reverse reaction in the TCA cycle. It is possible that other worms which excrete succinate (table 6.3) are obtaining energy in this manner.

## 6.3. *Energy metabolism during development*

The energy metabolism of the developmental stages of some parasitic worms often differs from that of their adult forms. The differences have probably evolved as the developmental stages have become adapted for growth and survival on a limited amount of endogenous or exogenous food in the presence of oxygen. This hypothesis may be illustrated by considering aspects of the development of *Ascaris*. The energy metabolism of unembryonated eggs of *Ascaris* appears to resemble that of the adult worms. In contrast, embryonation and development to the first and second larval stages within the egg shells do not occur in the absence of oxygen. The embryonating eggs contain a complete and functional electron transport system and the cyto-

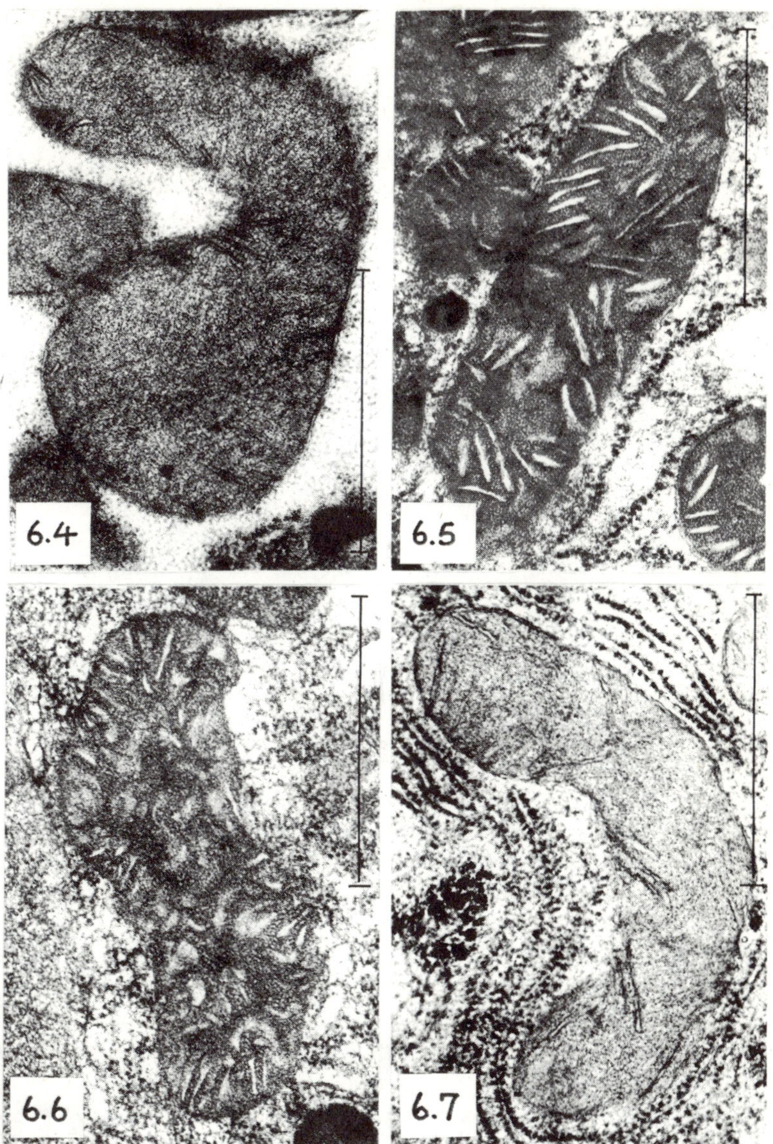


Figs. 6.4–6.7. Transmission electron micrographs of mitochondria from adult *Haemonchus contortus* and *Nippostrongylus brasiliensis* (Nematoda). The scales represent approximately 1 μm. 6.4 and 6.5 show mitochondria of different appearance from the same tissue (body wall muscle) of the same nematode (*Haemonchus*). 6.6 and 6.7 show mitochondria of different appearance from the same tissue (intestinal wall) of different nematodes (*Nippostrongylus* and *Haemonchus* respectively) (gift of E. A. Munn).

chromes are synthesized in response to oxygen. Development is bound to require much energy and the stored food reserves in the egg will obviously yield the maximum amount of energy if oxygen is used as the electron acceptor. The hatching of the infective eggs *in vitro* can occur anaerobically, and the parasites' energy metabolism reverts to that of the adult once it is established in its definitive host. The availability of oxygen is not the sole factor involved in this metabolic switch in the development of *Ascaris*. Adult *Ascaris* do not synthesize cytochromes on exposure to oxygen. The activities of the enzymes of the TCA cycle have also been demonstrated in preparations from eggs and larvae of *Ascaris*. Similar results have been obtained from larvae of *Haemonchus contortus, Strongyloides papillosus* and *Trichinella spiralis*, which also possess a complete electron transport system. These findings suggest that oxygen is of importance to the developing worms, but unequivocal proof is still awaited. A similar situation exists with regard to some of the developmental stages of certain digenean flukes and cestodes, but little information is available about developing acanthocephalan worms. It follows that fats and proteins will also be available for energy production (fig. 6.2) if developmental stages are able to utilize oxygen.

## 6.4. *Interactions between the energy metabolism of hosts and parasitic worms*

In vertebrates, the liver is a key organ in carbohydrate metabolism and it stores a substantial part of the body's reserve of glycogen. About 100 grams of carbohydrate is stored in the liver of a healthy, well-nourished man, in contrast to about 5 grams of glucose circulating in the blood. In the liver the glycogen is mobilized to maintain levels of blood sugar during fasting and stress, while at other times it is synthesized from glucose and other precursors. Several parasitic worms invade the livers of their hosts and much damage results from their presence. For example, immature *Fasciola* feed on liver cells and elicit an exaggerated host response, while the eggs of *Schistosoma* induce the development of lesions in the host's liver (9.2.3). *Fasciola* and other flukes occlude the ducts of the biliary system, and thus interfere with the clearance of toxic substances from the liver. It is difficult to imagine that the energy metabolism of a host is not impaired under such circumstances. Other parasitic worms affect the food intake, digestion and nutrient absorption of their hosts, whose energy metabolism is likely to be disturbed indirectly, especially if malnutrition or other forms of stress are evident.

At one time, intestinal worms were thought to consume a considerable part of the food eaten by the host. Even assuming that worms have very high metabolic rates, their mass compared with that of the host is usually negligible, and few calories would be lost to the worms from the host's daily intake. An infection of *Ascaris* from one person was found to weigh 5 kg, but the energy intake of so much worm tissue would probably not be more than about 8% of the 10500 kJ which are often ingested daily by well-fed individuals. In regions where the food supply is usually inadequate, however, a large worm burden of *Ascaris* may cause a serious loss of potential energy from the host. On the other hand, several of the excretory products of the energy metabolism of worms (table 6.3) could be degraded to release energy (fig. 6.2) if they were to be absorbed by the host's cells. The site of excretion of the volatile and non-volatile end-products of energy metabolism has been little studied. In *Ascaris*, the end-products appear to leave the worm in the faeces. In acanthocephalans, and probably also in tapeworms, loss through the tegument is likely to be important. A so-called excretory system has been described for flukes, tapeworms and nematodes, but little is known of its role in this context.

The developmental stages of digenean flukes usually lead to a decrease in the glycogen content of the invaded organs of molluscan hosts, compared with those from uninfected hosts. The average glycogen concentration in the digestive gland of uninfected male common periwinkles, *Littorina littorea*, was found to be $3.36 \pm 0.24$ mg per 100 mg wet weight of tissue. Similar periwinkles which were infected with developmental stages of the digenean *Cryptocotyle lingua* had an average glycogen concentration of $1.71 \pm 0.10$ mg per 100 mg wet weight of digestive gland.

## 6.5. *Energy metabolism and chemotherapy*

Research into the biochemistry of parasitic worms has been stimulated by man's need to control and cure parasitic infections in himself and in domestic animals. The main approach to chemotherapy is still an empirical one in which many compounds are synthesized and administered to infected animals in the hope that some anthelmintic activity will be detected. Recently another more rational approach to chemotherapy has developed in which the investigators seek to discover differences between the biochemistry of a parasite and its host. The aim is that the parasite should be vulnerable to chemotherapeutic attack without corresponding toxicity to the host. Irrespective of its mode of development, an ideal drug ought to have the following properties before it is offered for use. It should be safe and easy to administer and it should have a high therapeutic index, which is the ratio of toxic dose to effective dose. Its effect should be rapid, so that a short course of treatment is needed, and it should not accumulate in the host's tissues. It should not induce drug resistance on the part of the parasite. It should be synthetic so that identical batches can be prepared, and it should be stable under a wide range of storage conditions. Finally it needs to be cheap, so that the people who require it can afford to buy it. The costs of chemotherapeutic research, safety tests, clinical trials, advertising and marketing are enormous. Nevertheless, some progress is being made in the chemotherapy of worm infections. The reactions leading to the formation of

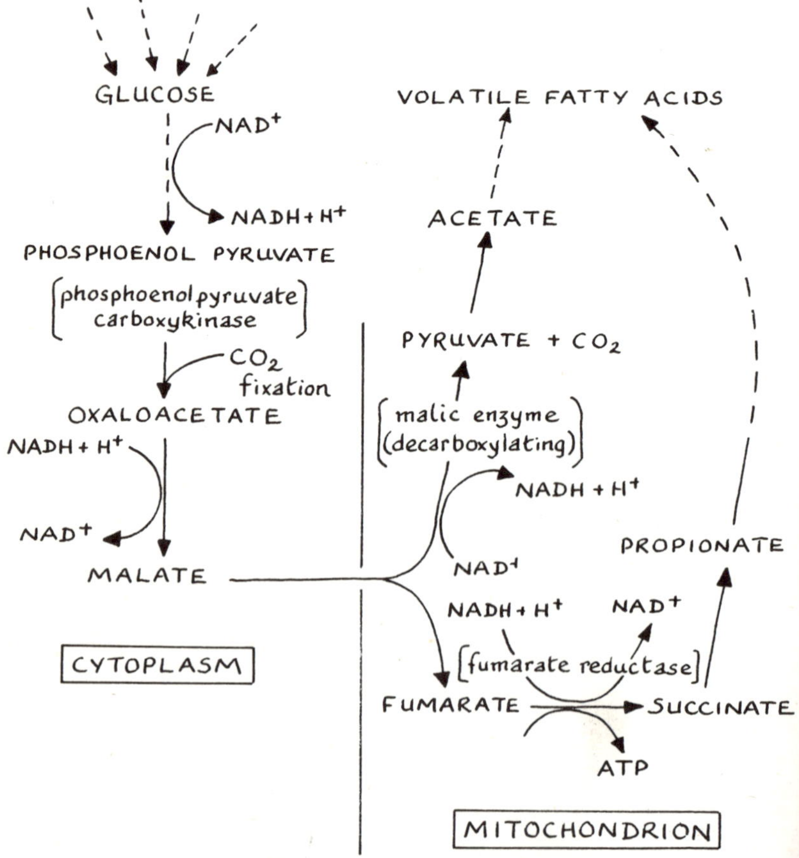


Fig. 6.8. A flow diagram showing the probable route of carbohydrate catabolism in the muscle of adult *Ascaris* (Nematoda) (after Saz, 1972).

ATP in the mitochondria of *Ascaris* and the excretion of succinate (fig. 6.8) do not occur in mammals. Unfortunately, the synthesis of a specific enzyme inhibitor, or any compound which might interfere with a metabolic pathway, is as time-consuming and tedious as the routine screening of numerous new compounds. In the case of *Ascaris*, however, empirical screening and biochemical research have developed tetramisole (generic name for the hydrochloride of 2,3,5,6-tetrahydro-6-phenyl-imidazo(2,1B)thiazole), the laevo isomer of which inhibits the fumarate-succinate system of the worm (fig. 6.8). Particulate preparations of *Ascaris* muscle produce ATP *in vitro* in the presence of malate, ADP and inorganic phosphate. Addition of L-tetramisole to the system results in a decreased incorporation of phosphate into ATP, presumably because the drug has interfered with the activity of fumarate reductase (fig. 6.8). Administration of the drug to people infected with *Ascaris* is quickly followed by the expulsion of the worms, which are seen to be alive, but immobilized. Paralysis is to be expected if a major energy-yielding reaction of the worm's muscles has been blocked. Other anthelmintic drugs, which interfere with the production of energy from carbohydrate, are currently in use.

# 7. Reproduction

Most parasitic flatworms are protandrous hermaphrodites, in which the male organs mature before those of the female. All known acanthocephalans are dioecious, as are most nematodes. Some exceptions to these generalizations have been cited in Chapter 1, others will be mentioned below and no doubt more will be discovered as our knowledge increases. Usually, fertilized eggs are the end-products of sexual reproduction. The term 'egg' is used by parasitologists to include various stages from a very early embryo to advanced larval forms enclosed within complex egg shells (figs. 3.1–3.16).

The basic features of the reproductive systems of parasitic worms have been illustrated in figs. 1.4, 1.8, 1.22–1.24, 1.38, 1.39, 1.47 and 1.50. Species of monogenean and digenean flukes usually possess a single ovary and 1, 2 or 3 testes. Each proglottis of a tapeworm generally contains one ovary, but the number of testes per mature proglottis varies between species and has thus become an important taxonomic feature. There are 3 testes per proglottis of *Hymenolepis* and between 750 and 800 per proglottis of *Diphyllobothrium latum*. Male acanthocephalans usually have 2 testes, although some species, for example *Moniliformis*, have occasional males with only 1; such individuals, called monorchic, are known to function normally in reproduction. The female reproductive system of acanthocephalans is unique. The primordial ovarian tissue of the developing female gives rise to separate ovaries, which are often termed ovarian balls (fig. 1.38). These in turn give rise to more ovarian balls and the process continues until large numbers have been formed. About 7 are present in a one-week-old female *Moniliformis* and over 6000 are present some weeks later. The ovarian balls are contained in the fluid of the body cavity either floating freely or loosely constrained in membranous chambers known as ligament sacs.

Most male nematodes have one testis, and most females have two ovaries. Towards the end of the 19th century, observations on the reproduction of *Ascaris* made a major contribution to genetics and embryology; it was discovered that equal amounts of nuclear material came from the egg and the sperm during fertilization, and the developmental fate of cells during the early stages of cleavage in the embryo was traced. Earlier in the same century, even the most expert biologist was likely to embrace the doctrine of spontaneous generation of parasitic worms.

## 7.1. *Prepatent and patent periods*

The prepatent period is the time which elapses between the establishment of a worm on or in its definitive host and the release of the first eggs. The patent period is the extent of the time of egg release. During the prepatent period, the worms grow and often change site in their hosts. Their gonads and gametes develop and insemination occurs for the first time. Many factors are known to affect both the prepatent and patent periods, including the innate properties and longevity of the worms, the structure of the worm population, the nutritional, physiological and immunological status of the host and the other organisms which are also present in the host. These factors also affect the numbers of eggs which are produced by individual worms and populations of worms, and the asexual aspects of reproduction.

Some estimates of the egg production of parasitic worms have been given in table 3.1. It is unlikely that general agreement would be found about the egg production of a given worm. Figures for the egg production of individual female *Ascaris* in pigs have been variously quoted as 200000 eggs daily (table 3.1), 1.4 million eggs daily and nearly 2 million eggs daily. This last estimate was obtained as follows. A naturally infected pig was isolated as soon as eggs of *Ascaris* were detected in its faeces. Twice daily thereafter, samples of the pig's faeces were collected and the number of eggs per gram of faeces was determined. The total egg output for a 24 hour period was obtained by multiplying the average of the two counts by the number of grammes of faeces passed by the pig during the period. The pig was constantly moved to a clean pen in an attempt to reduce the chances of its acquiring further infections of *Ascaris*. When egg production stopped, the figures calculated for total daily egg output were related to the number of worms present in the pig. On average, a female *Ascaris* appeared to produce approximately 2 million eggs per 24 hours. In addition, the patent period of the worm was found to be about 50 weeks.

The survival and successful transmission of *Ascaris* between hosts is linked to the production of many specialized eggs per day for about a year (see Chapter 3). The survival of monogenean flukes of the genus *Gyrodactylus* is achieved by an equally specialized, but different, method which depends on viviparty. *Gyrodactylus elegans*, from the gills of European freshwater fish, forms a zygote which does not acquire egg shells, but develops into an embryo within the body of the parent. Before the embryo is born, it has already given rise to another embryo within itself, and this in turn to another smaller embryo, which may contain a fourth and smallest embryo. The manner in which a population of *Gyrodactylus* could develop from one fluke during 20 days is shown in fig. 7.1. As in mammals, viviparity is linked with a decrease in the numbers of offspring, each of which appears to have a much better chance of survival.

## 7.2. *Mating behaviour*

Very little is known about the manner in which male and female worms, or cross-inseminating hermaphrodites, find their partners during the prepatent period. Several experiments have been performed in which male and female worms have been placed by surgical techniques in different locations in a host. After a given time, examination of the host has shown that the worms have come into contact and that insemination has occurred. The hookworm *Ancylostoma caninum* and the acanthocephalan *Moniliformis* appear to be able to find partners after surgical transfer. The digenean fluke *Paragonimus kellicotti* usually lives with a hermaphroditic partner in a cyst in the lungs of cats. When cats are infected experimentally with a single metacercaria of *P. kellicotti*, fertile eggs are not produced, but when cats which have received one metacercaria are given a second 8 weeks after the first, two flukes are eventually retrieved from the same cyst and reproduction is found to have occurred.

Experiments conducted *in vitro* have suggested that nematodes respond to attractant chemicals released by their own kind. In *Trichinella spiralis* and *Aspiculuris tetraptera*, the two sexes have been found to be attractive to each other when they are separated in chambers designed to allow chemical contact through water-borne molecules. The males and females of some species of worm remain in very close contact after they have found each other. Adult blood flukes live in pairs in the blood vessels of their hosts. The small male of the nematode *Trichosomoides crassicauda*, which inhabits the bladder of the rat, enters and often remains in the female worm's vagina. The monogenean fluke *Diplozoon paradoxum* apparently becomes permanently attached to its partner. After a larval *D. paradoxum* has become attached to the gills of a suitable host, a small

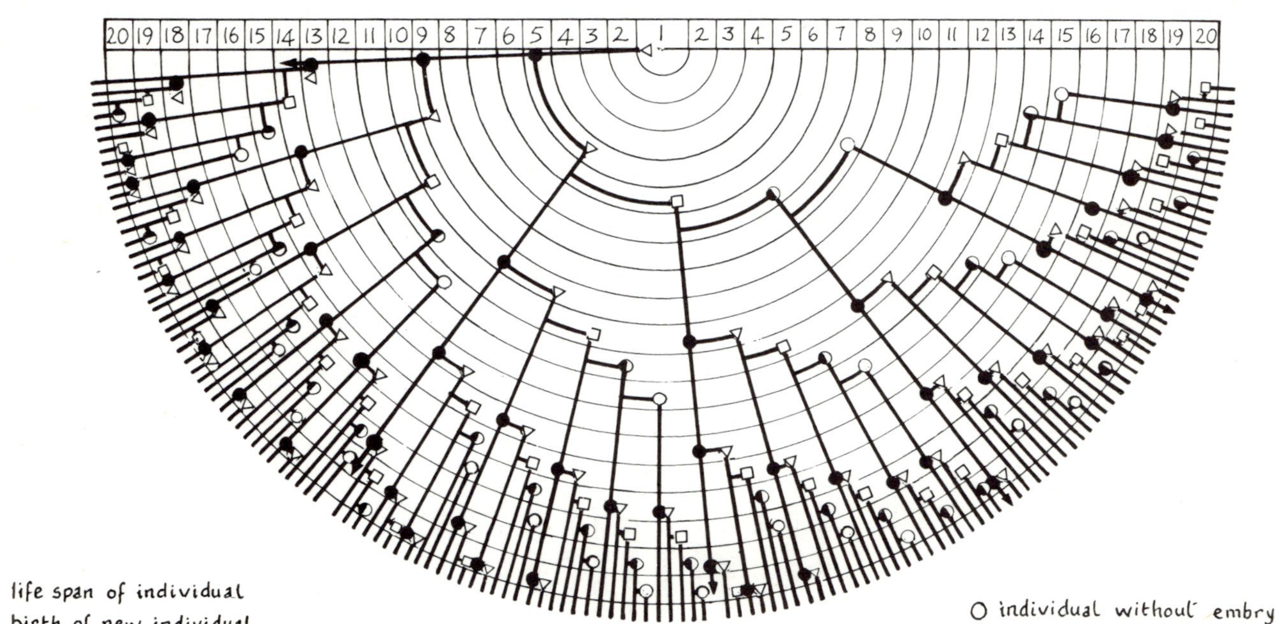


Fig. 7.1. Diagram showing the increase in progeny from an individual *Gyrodactylus* (Monogenea) during 20 days (after Bychowsky, 1957, *Monogenetic Trematodes*).

sucker develops in the middle of its ventral surface and a conical process on its dorsal surface (fig. 7.2). Two individuals come together and the ventral sucker of one grasps the dorsal cone of the other. The young worms then twist so that the male pore of one becomes closely opposed to the vaginal pore of the other and *vice versa*. The remaining free mid-ventral sucker grips the free dorsal cone and the linked worms mature and remain in this position (fig. 7.3).

## 7.3. *Copulation and insemination*

### 7.3.1. *Hermaphrodites*

In theory, most species of parasitic platyhelminth may reproduce sexually, either by self or cross-insemination, or by both methods. Copulation has rarely been observed, but flukes appear to adopt particular positions (fig. 7.4) and the sperm are assumed to be transferred by means of the cirrus or other intromittent apparatus (see fig. 1.7). In some flukes, cross-insemination appears to be the usual practice. The nuclei of sperms in the eye fluke, *Philophthalmus megalurus*, were labelled *in vitro* with $^3$H-thymidine. Marked individual worms were returned to the eyes of chicks, some of which contained small populations of unmarked worms. After an appropriate time the worms were recovered and the location of the radioactive label was determined by autoradiography. Twenty-eight of 37 marked worms inseminated themselves when no partners were available, whereas only 1 worm out of 33 marked worms inseminated itself when other worms were present. The tendency for young worms to inseminate themselves increased when old worms were present in the host. The monogenean fluke *Diplectanum aequans*, which lives on the gills of bass, is interesting and unusual in that the sperm are transferred by means of a spermatophore. The spermatophores are shaped like an internal cast of the penis, which is used to deposit the spermatophore during copulation.

Various theories have been advanced to explain how insemination is carried out by tapeworms. Self-fertilization could occur by the eversion of the cirrus into the vagina of the same proglottis or by the insertion of cirri from anterior proglottides into the vagina of posterior proglottides (figs. 1.22–1.24). The protandrous nature of gonadial development in tapeworms would favour this latter method of self-insemination. There is also the possibility that sperm may be emitted into the fluid environment of the worm, from which they could swim into the female reproductive tract. In fact, both self and cross-insemination occur in tapeworms, and copulation is involved.

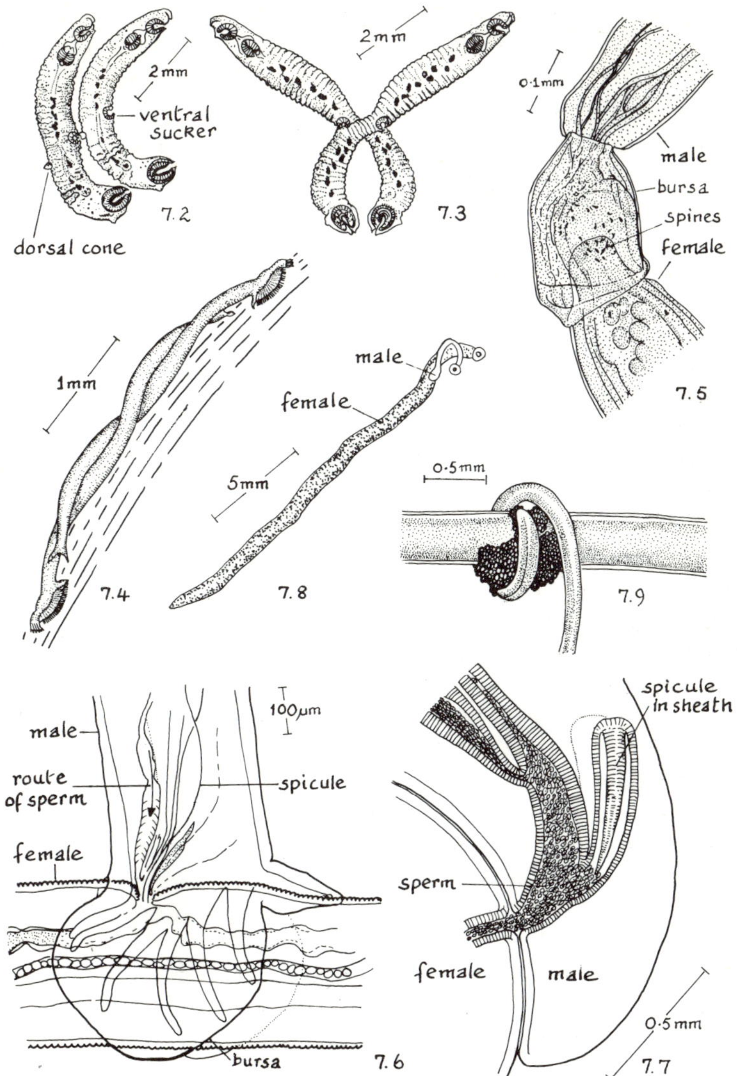


Figs. 7.2–7.9. Aspects of mating in parasitic worms. 7.2. Coming together of *Diplozoon paradoxum* (Monogenea). 7.3. Paired *D. paradoxum* (after Zeder, 1872). 7.4. *Macrogyrodactylus polypteri* (Monogenea) *in copula* (after Malmberg, 1957, *Arch. f. Zool.*, **10**, 317). 7.5. *Gorgorhynchus clavatum* (Acanthocephala) *in copula* (after Yamaguti, 1963, *Systema Helminthum. V. Acanthocephala*). 7.6. *Ancylostoma* sp. (Nematoda) *in copula* (after Muller, 1975, *Worms and Disease*). 7.7. Section through *Ascaris lumbricoides* (Nematoda) *in copula* (after Mueller, 1930, *Trans Am. microsc. Soc.*, **49**, 42). 7.8. *Syngamus trachea* (Nematoda) *in copula* (after Lapage, 1968, *Veterinary Parasitology*, 2nd. edn.). 7.9. *Mermis subnigrescens* (Nematoda) *in copula* (after Christie, 1937, *J. agric. Res.*, **55**, 353).

Histological preparations have clearly revealed the cirrus of a proglottis of *Phyllobothrium sinuosiceps* inserted into the vagina of the same proglottis. Similar preparations have shown the cirrus from a proglottis of a strobila of *Acanthobothrium quadripartitum* in the vagina of another individual's proglottis whose cirrus was in the vagina of a third tapeworm. Tapeworms of the family Acoleidae lack vaginal openings and insemination may occur by thrusting the armoured cirrus directly through the tegument.

### 7.3.2. *Dioecious species*

A male acanthocephalan is equipped with an eversible copulatory bursa which is an extension of the worm's body wall (fig. 1.39). When copulation occurs, the bursa enfolds the posterior end of the female (fig. 7.5) into which sperm are discharged, presumably by means of the penis. The posterior ends of some species of acanthocephalan are equipped with small spines which may help to keep the worms together during copulation (fig. 1.44). Male acanthocephalans also possess characteristic cement glands. Possibly the secretions of the cement glands block the female's vagina for long enough to prevent the loss of sperm.

Information about copulation and insemination in acanthocephalans has been obtained from experimental infections of *Moniliformis*. Individual male worms were introduced into the small intestine of rats, together with varying numbers of unmated females. The maximum number of females a single male was capable of inseminating was found to be 17. None of these females reached its full capacity for egg production or experienced a complete patent period. The egg production of females was also curtailed when their contact with males was restricted to the first 5 weeks of the infection. Copulation and insemination could take place during this early phase of the infection, for evidence for the occurrence of these events has been obtained as early as 16 days after the start of the infection. It is likely, therefore, that *Moniliformis* copulates several times before sufficient sperms are transferred for the fertilization of the available female gametes. It is not known for how long sperms can be stored in a female acanthocephalan, although they can be seen swimming in fresh samples of fluid from the body cavities of inseminated females.

The males of most species of nematode are equipped with spicules, and in addition may possess a copulatory bursa (figs. 7.6, 7.7). The spicules are usually inserted into the female during copulation, but their function has not been fully resolved. The left spicule of *Proleptus obtusus* is longer than the right and serves to channel the flow of sperm from the male to the female. In contrast, a pair of *Ascaris* have been fixed *in copula* with no sign of spicule participation (fig. 7.7). The bursa of a male nematode may be sensitive to substances released from or near the vulva of a female of the same species. The position of copulation depends on the location of the female's vulva or genital pore (fig. 1.50). In *Ancylostoma* spp., *Syngamus trachea* and *Mermis subnigrescens* (figs. 7.6, 7.8, 7.9), the vulva is not terminal and the male grips the female's body at right angles to his own. In *Nematospiroides dubius*, the female's vulva is at the posterior end and the worms lie with their heads directed in opposite directions during copulation; a colourless substance, which is secreted by the copulatory glands of the male, is transferred to the females in addition to sperm. Presumably the sperm of all species of parasitic worm are bathed in some form of seminal fluid. Their sperm have been found to contain glycogen, but it is not known whether endogenous reserves are sufficient for their survival in female worms or whether exogenous nutrients are needed; the sperm of *Ancylostoma caninum* may live for as long as three weeks in the female worm's reproductive tract.

## 7.4. *Spermatogenesis*

Studies of many animals, including parasitic worms, have established that the production of spermatozoa in the testes (a process called spermatogenesis) may be considered in three phases. In the first, spermatocytogenesis occurs, in which the spermatogonia proliferate by mitotic division to give rise to spermatocytes. In the second, the spermatocytes undergo meiotic reduction divisions to produce clusters of spermatids containing the haploid number of chromosomes. In the third phase, known as spermiogenesis, the spermatids undergo a remarkable series of cytological transformations leading to the formation of the sperm.

Each spermatogonium of the monogenean fluke, *Diclidophora merlangi*, gives rise by mitosis to 4 spermatogonia which, in turn, divide to form a group of 8 primary spermatocytes. Cytoplasmic bridges link the spermatocytes and the meiotic phase of spermatogenesis produces a rosette of 32 spermatids from which the sperm develop. The different cell types involved can be seen in a tissue section of a testis of *D. merlangi* (fig. 7.10). Spermatogenesis in digenean flukes, tapeworms, acanthocephalans and nematodes occurs in more or less the same fashion, but there are some differences of detail. For example, rosettes of 64 spermatids are formed in certain tapeworms; during spermiogenesis in acanthocephalans and nematodes, the nuclear envelope disintegrates and the nuclear and cytoplasmic components intermingle.

Structural features of the sperm of parasitic worms are shown in figs. 7.12 to 7.23. The sperm of many animals have an acrosome (fig. 7.11) which is known to be involved in the penetration of the egg. Unusually, the sperm of parastic worms studied so far appear to lack an acrosome. The sperm of monogenean and digenean flukes are usually filariform in shape and in cross section two axial filaments can be seen (fig. 7.14); each has a 9+1 fibre configuration compared with the familiar 9+2 of mammalian sperm tails (fig. 7.11). In contrast a single axial filament is present in the sperm of tapeworms (fig. 7.19). Acanthocephalan sperm are also filariform, but the axial filament of the tail may or may not have the 9+2 configuration (fig. 7.20). During spermiogenesis in *Polymorphus minutus*, the mitochondria of the spermatids are excluded from the sperm. Nevertheless, the sperm can be seen to be active and motile *in vitro*. The sperm of nematodes

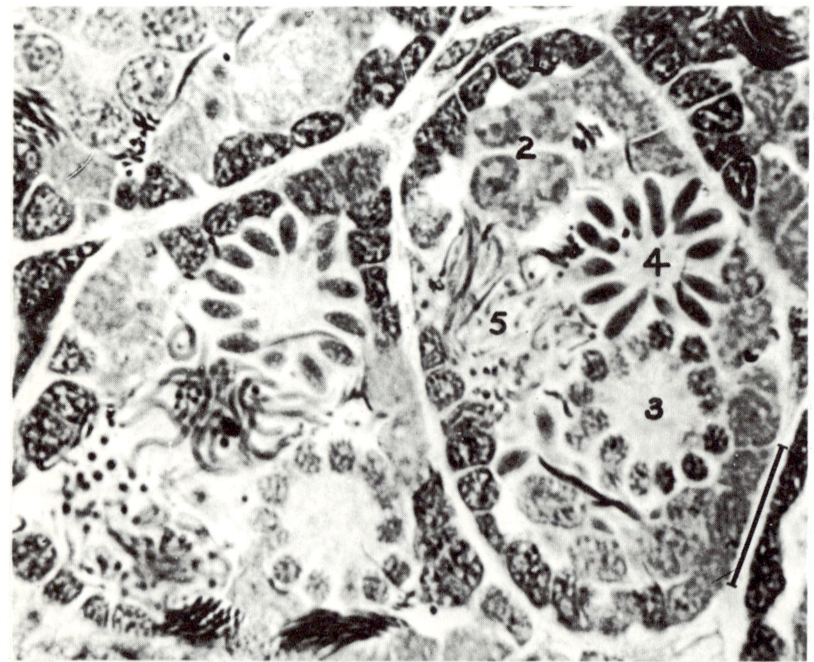


Fig. 7.10. Photomicrograph of a section through the testis of *Diclidophora merlangi* (Monogenea) showing the following stages of spermatogenesis: spermatogonia (1), spermatocytes (2), rosettes of spermatids (3 and 4) and spermatozoa (5). The scale represents approximately 25 $\mu$m. (from Halton and Hardcastle, 1976, *Int. J. Parasit.*, **6**, 43).

are very different from those of other types of parasitic worms (figs. 7.21–7.23). Those of *Ascaris* (fig. 7.22) are amoeboid in appearance, and pseudopodia have been seen to extend from their surfaces. Similar extensions have been observed from the sperm of *Aspiculuris tetraptera* (fig. 7.23). The nucleic acid of the sperm of *A. tetraptera* and *N. brasiliensis* (fig. 7.21) is located in the tail-like structure; the term 'tail-like' has to be used since neither these structures nor the entire sperm of either species have been observed to move *in vitro*.

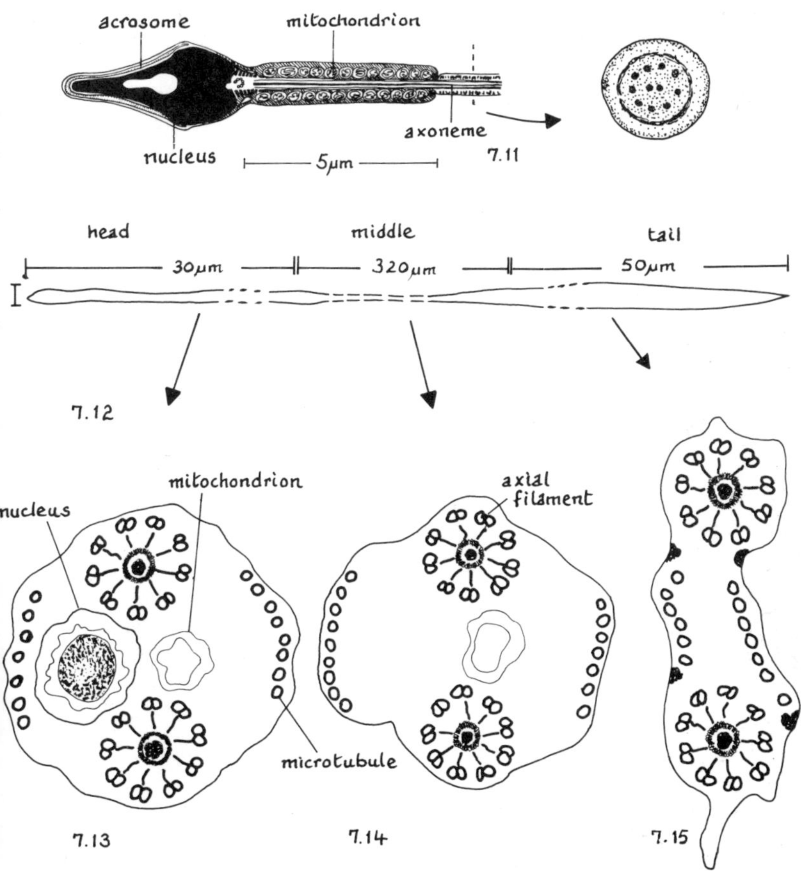


Figs 7.11–7.15. Spermatozoan structure. 7.11. Diagram of a sagittal section through a human spermatozoon (after Baccetti and Afzelius, 1976, *The Biology of the Sperm Cell*). 7.12. Spermatozoon of *Haematoloechus medioplexus* (Digenea). 7.13–7.15. Diagrammatic reconstructions, based on electron micrographs, of transverse sections through the head, middle and tail regions of a spermatozoon of *H. medioplexus* (after Burton, 1972, *J. Parasit.*, **58**, 68).

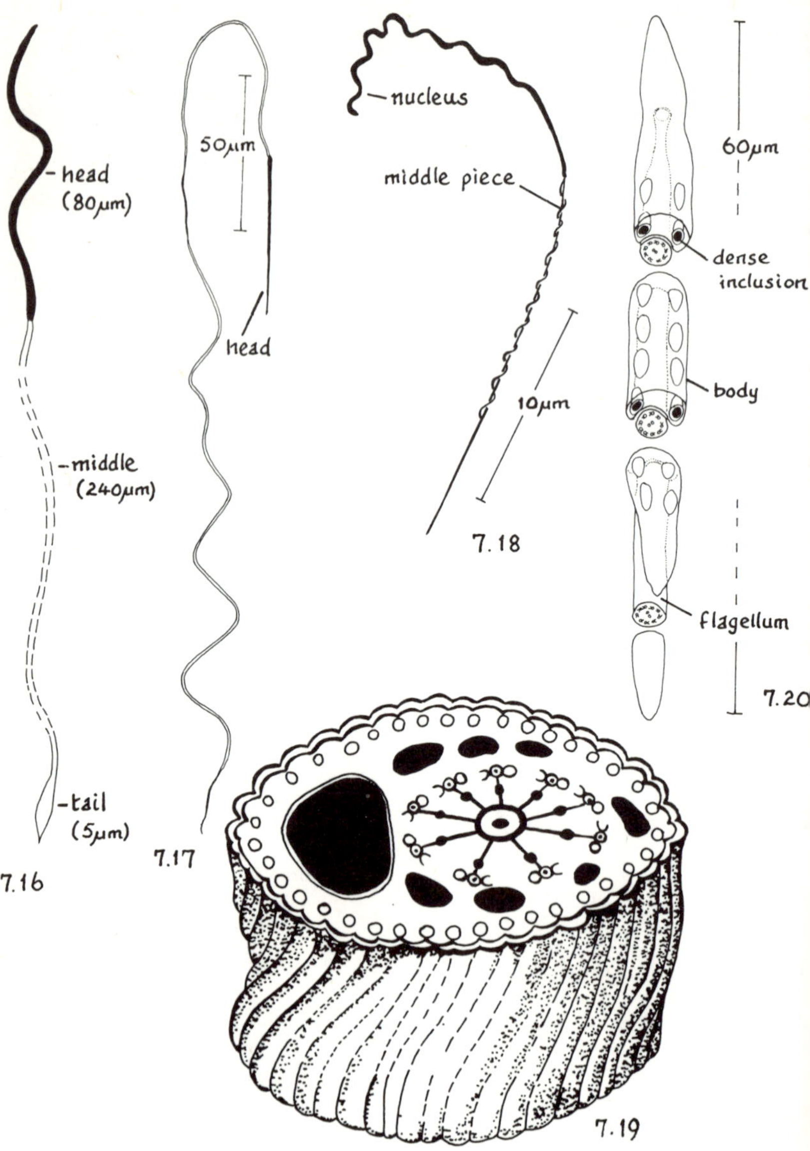


Figs. 7.16–7.20. Spermatozoan structure. 7.16. *Diclidophora merlangi* (Monogenea) (after Halton and Hardcastle, 1976, *Int. J. Parasit.*, **6**, 43). 7.17. *Fasciola hepatica* (Digenea) (after Hendelberg, 1962, *Zool. Bdrg. Uppsala*, **35**, 569). 7.18. *Baerietta diana* (Cestoda) (after Rybicka, 1966, *Adv. Parasit.*, **4**, 107). 7.19. Diagrammatic reconstruction of a segment of a spermatozoon of *Moniezia expansa* (Cestoda) (after Swiderski, 1968, *Zool. Pol.*, **18**, 475). 7.20. *Polymorphus minutus* (Acanthocephala) (after Whitfield, 1971, *Parasitology*, **62**, 415).

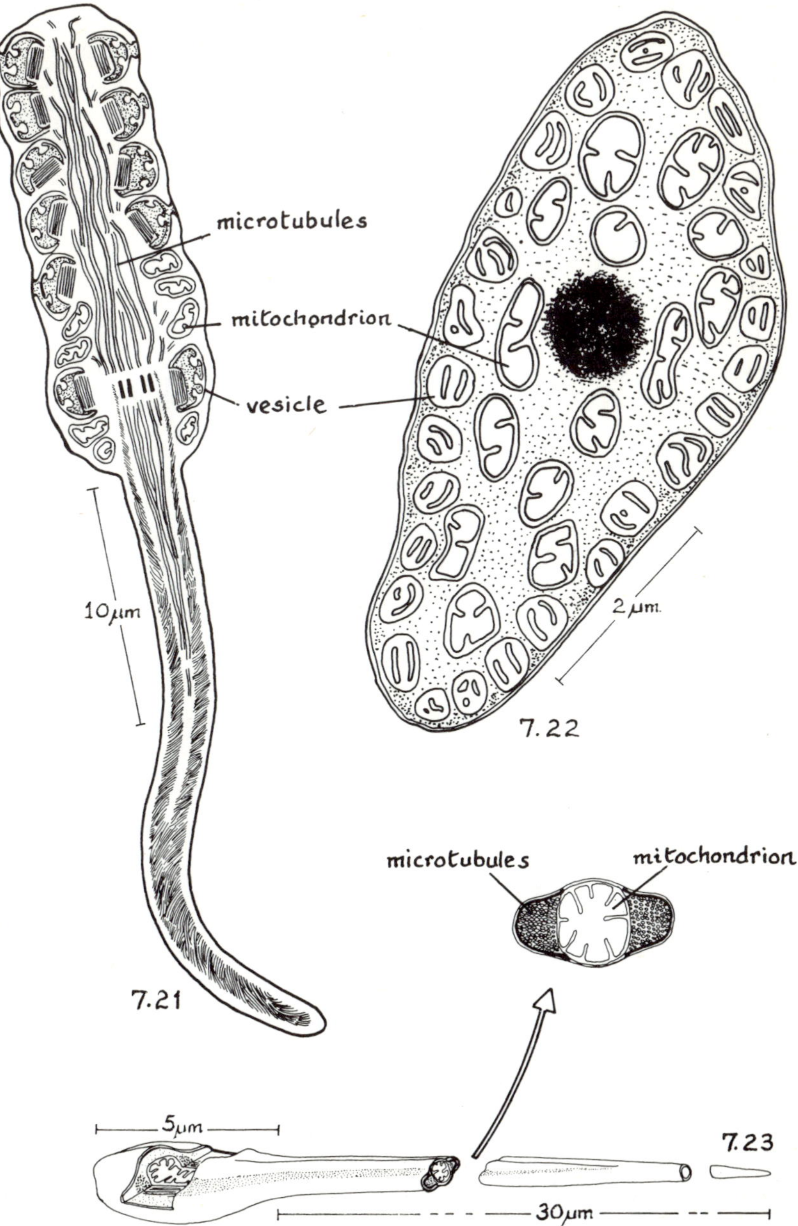


Figs. 7.21–7.23. Nematode spermatozoan structure. 7.21. *Nippostrongylus brasiliensis* (after Jamuar, 1966, *J. Cell. Biol.*, **31**, 381). 7.22. *Ascaris lumbricoides* (after Bird, 1971). 7.23. *Aspiculuris tetraptera* (after Lee and Anya, 1967, *J. Cell Sci.*, **2**, 537).

## 7.5. *Oogenesis*

Oogenesis is the process whereby the primordial germ-cells of the ovary are transformed into the mature oocytes or egg-cells. Usually, the division of primordial germ cells produces oogonia, each of which may grow and become a primary oocyte. In many animals, the primary oocyte divides by meiosis to form a haploid secondary oocyte and polar bodies. Fertilization may now take place or, as happens in several parasitic worms, a sperm may penetrate a developing oocyte and thus stimulate the completion of the meiotic division and the formation of the polar bodies.

Oogenesis is a very interesting process in the acanthocephalans *Moniliformis* and *Polymorphus minutus*. The mature ovarian ball consists of an oogonial syncytium and a cellular zone, both of which are embedded in a supporting syncytium (fig. 7.24). A portion of cytoplasm containing a nucleus becomes detached from the oogonial syncytium. This cell now constitutes an oogonium which divides mitotically to form primary oocytes. Eventually, these become the mature oocytes orientated in the peripheral region of the ovarian ball (fig. 7.24). Thus, the number of nuclei in the oogonial syncytia of all the ovarian balls of a mature female acanthocephalan is a measure of the egg-producing potential of the worm.

Syncytial tissue is also involved in oogenesis in *Ascaris*. The reproductive tract of a female *Ascaris* is shown in fig. 7.25. The oogonia arise at the distal or blind ends of the paired, elongated ovaries. In section, the oogonia in this region appear as portions of nucleated cytoplasm united by a common stalk running the length of this part of the ovary. The change of these oogonia to primary and mature oocytes occurs as the tissue develops along the linearly expanded ovary. At the end of their journey, the mature oocytes, which have by now acquired relatively large quantities of carbohydrate, lipid and protein, become detached from the stalk and fall into the oviduct where fertilization occurs.

## 7.6. *Fertilization*

The few observations which have been made to date on fertilization in parasitic worms appear to fit into the current concept of the process in free-living animals. The main events of fertilization are the interaction between the sperm and the egg before contact is established between them, their interaction following the establishment of physical contact, and the activation of the egg after the penetration of the sperm. The final event involves the fusion of the nuclei and the initiation of development. The manner in which some

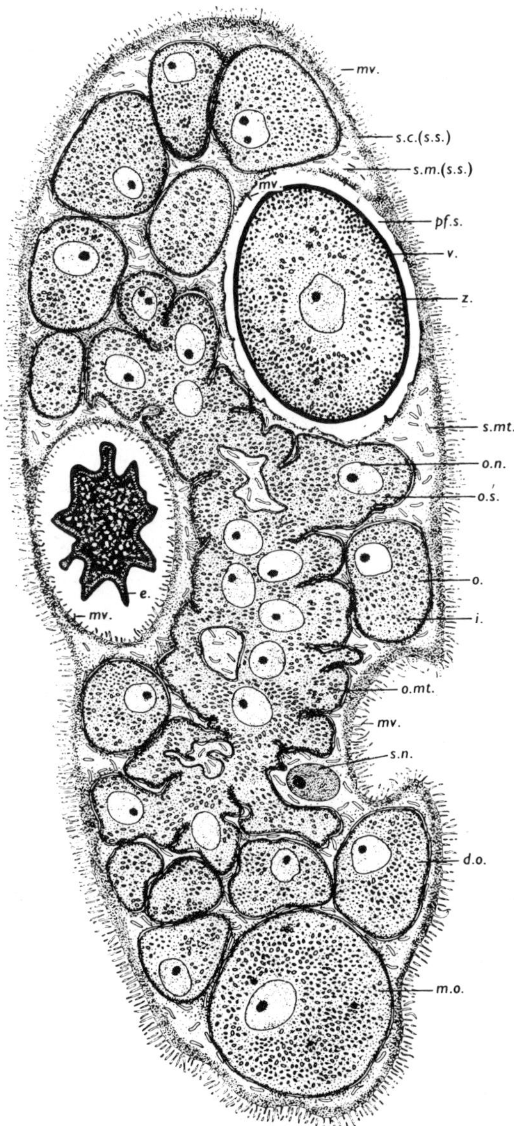


Fig. 7.24. Diagrammatic representation of the organization of an ovarian ball from an inseminated female *Moniliformis dubius* (Acanthocephala). *d.o.*, developing oocyte; *e.*, egg; *i.*, inclusion; *mv.*, microvillus; *m.o.*, mature oocyte; *o.*, oogonium; *o.mt.*, mitochondria; *o.n.*, nucleus; *o.s.*, oogonial syncytium; *pf.s.*, post-fertilization space; *s.c.*, cortex; *s.m.*, medulla; *s.mt.*, mitochondrion; *s.n.*, nucleus; *s.s.*, supporting syncytium; *v.*, vitelline membrane and *z.*, zygote (from Crompton and Whitfield, 1974, *Parasitology*, **69**, 429).

of these events are achieved in worms is different from that in free-living animals; perhaps the differences are to be expected if the structures of the sperm are different (see figs. 7.11–7.23).

In parasitic flatworms, fertilization occurs in the part of the reproductive tract known as the ootype (fig. 7.26). The membrane of the active sperm of the lung fluke *Haematoloechus medioplexus* fuses with the membrane of the egg-cell and thus both cells become one (fig. 7.27). This act of fertilization results in a considerable increase in the volume of the egg, which may have received a large quantity of nutrients in the form of the sperm, in addition to the hereditary material. The sperm of the tapeworm *Baerietta diana* (fig. 7.18) coils around the mature egg, but only the head passes into the cell while the middle and tail pieces remain outside.

After copulation between acanthocephalan worms, the sperm move up the female reproductive tract and are assumed to reach the body cavity through openings in the uterine bell (fig. 7.28). The sperm are now in the vicinity of the ovarian balls, and some sperm pass through the cortical region of the supporting syncytium of the ovarian ball and penetrate the mature oocytes (fig. 7.24). Electron micrographs of

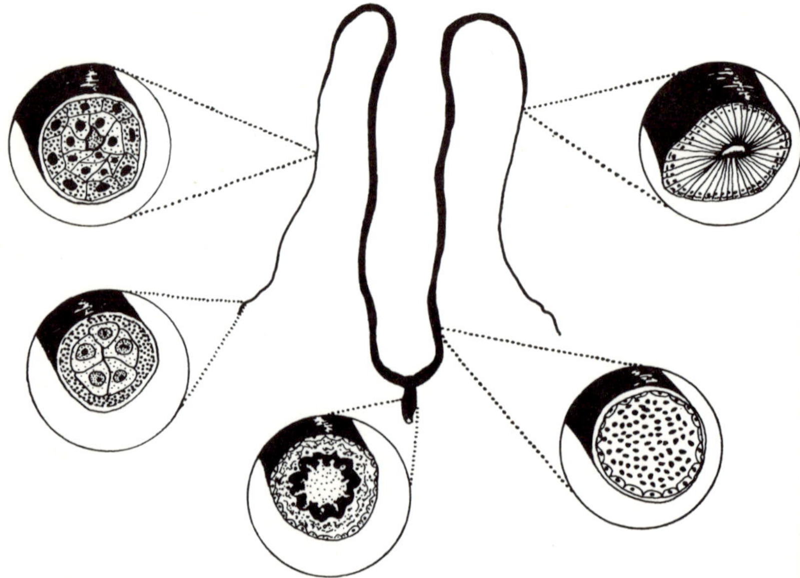

Fig. 7.25. Simplified representation of the female reproductive system of *Ascaris lumbricoides* (Nematoda) showing sections of the tract at various points (after Harris and Crofton, 1958, *New Biology*, 27).

ovarian balls in *Polymorphus* suggest that a whole sperm may enter the mature oocyte during fertilization. Sperm of the filarial nematode *Dipetalonema viteae* appear to be elongated when they leave the male worm, but they have been observed to be spherical in shape in the reproductive tract of the female. Similar changes in the shape of the sperm of *Nematospiroides dubius* have been observed, and those involved in fertilization are probably the globular variety. Perhaps these changes indicate that the sperms of parasitic worms cannot function without some contribution from the female reproductive

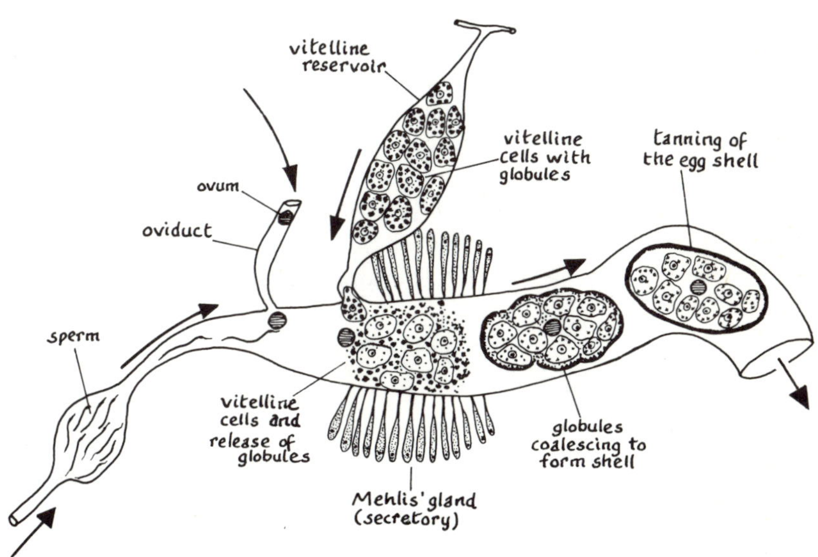


Fig. 7.26. Diagrammatic representation of eggshell formation in the ootype of a cestode (after Smyth, 1956, *Exptl Parasit.*, **5**, 519).

tract. As in the other species of parasitic worm, the single sperm that first enters the egg initiates changes that prevent the entry of other sperms. Other metabolic events accompany fertilization including the synthesis of ribosomes in the cytoplasm of the zygote.

Eggs of the digenean flukes *Coitacaecum anaspidis* and *Zygocotyle lunata* and the nematode *Mermis subnigrescens* can develop parthenogenetically without the intervention of sperm. Miracidia of parthenogenetic origin in *Z. lunata* are not as infective to snails as the miracidia from fertile eggs. Single-sex infections of the blood fluke *Schistosomatium douthitti* have been established experimentally in rodents; eggs containing miracidia have been obtained from female worms which had not had any contact with males. The miracidia were infective to snails, and cercariae eventually developed, but these were less infective to definitive hosts than cercariae which arose from fertile eggs.

## 7.7. *Development of eggshells and release of eggs*

### 7.7.1. *Development of eggshells*

The formation of the complex eggshells is usually an immediate consequence of fertilization. In most species of parasitic platyhelminth, the newly formed zygote is joined by a characteristic number of vitelline cells in the ootype (fig. 7.26). For example, 5 to 7 vitelline cells are involved in egg development in *Clonorchis* sp. and about 30 in *Fasciola*. The vitelline cells contain a variety of granules, and as the formation of the eggshells proceeds the number of granules in the cells appears to decrease. Eventually, the zygote is encased in the completed shell with the remains of the vitelline cells which might possibly serve as a supply of nutrients. While zygote and vitelline cells are being gathered together, secretions from other components of the ootype are also available for incorporation into the eggshells. The

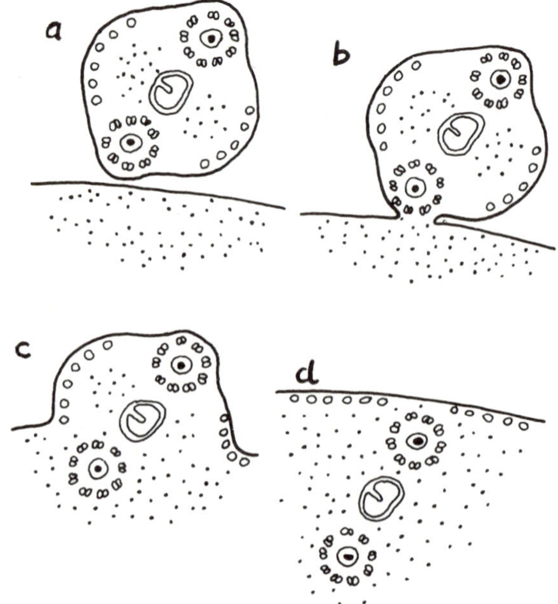


Fig. 7.27. An interpretation of the sequence of events (a–d) occurring during the fusion of the gametes of *Haematoloechus medioplexus* (Digenea) (after Burton, 1967, *J. Parasit.*, **53**, 994).

eggs of some flukes and cestodes (figs. 3.3, 3.4) are equipped with an operculum through which the larva escapes on hatching. The simplified scheme of eggshell formation shown in fig. 7.26 does not explain how an operculum or various projections (fig. 3.5) are formed.

The formation of the shell of an acanthocephalan egg begins while the zygote is still part of an ovarian ball (fig. 7.24) and continues while the egg is free in the body cavity. The materials for eggshell formation are assumed to be provided by substances present in the mature oocytes and in the body fluid. Eventually, the female body cavity contains eggs in all stages of development from young zygotes to shelled acanthors, but it is usually only the infective stages which pass into the uterus and out of the worm. The sorting of the eggs appears to occur in the uterine bell (fig. 7.28) in the manner suggested in fig. 7.29. The need to separate mature from immature eggs before release from the parent does not arise in platyhelminths where eggshell formation occurs in a production line, with the completion of

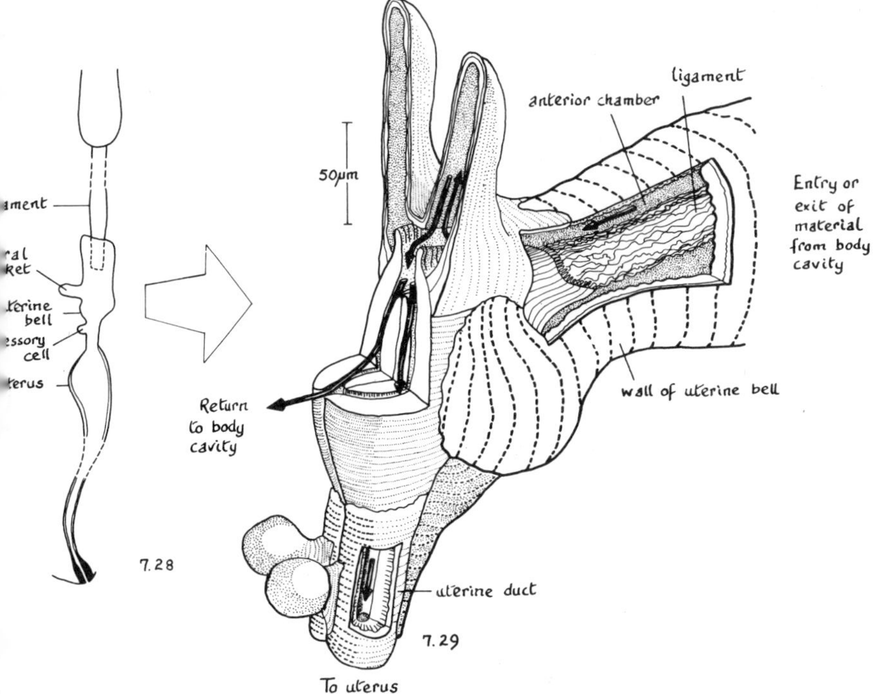


Figs. 7.28 and 7.29. Aspects of the female reproductive system of *Polymorphus minutus* (Acanthocephala). 7.28. Main components of the system. 7.29. Stereogram of a functional uterine bell in which possible routes for egg translocation are indicated by heavy arrows (after Whitfield, 1968, *Parasitology*, **58**, 671).

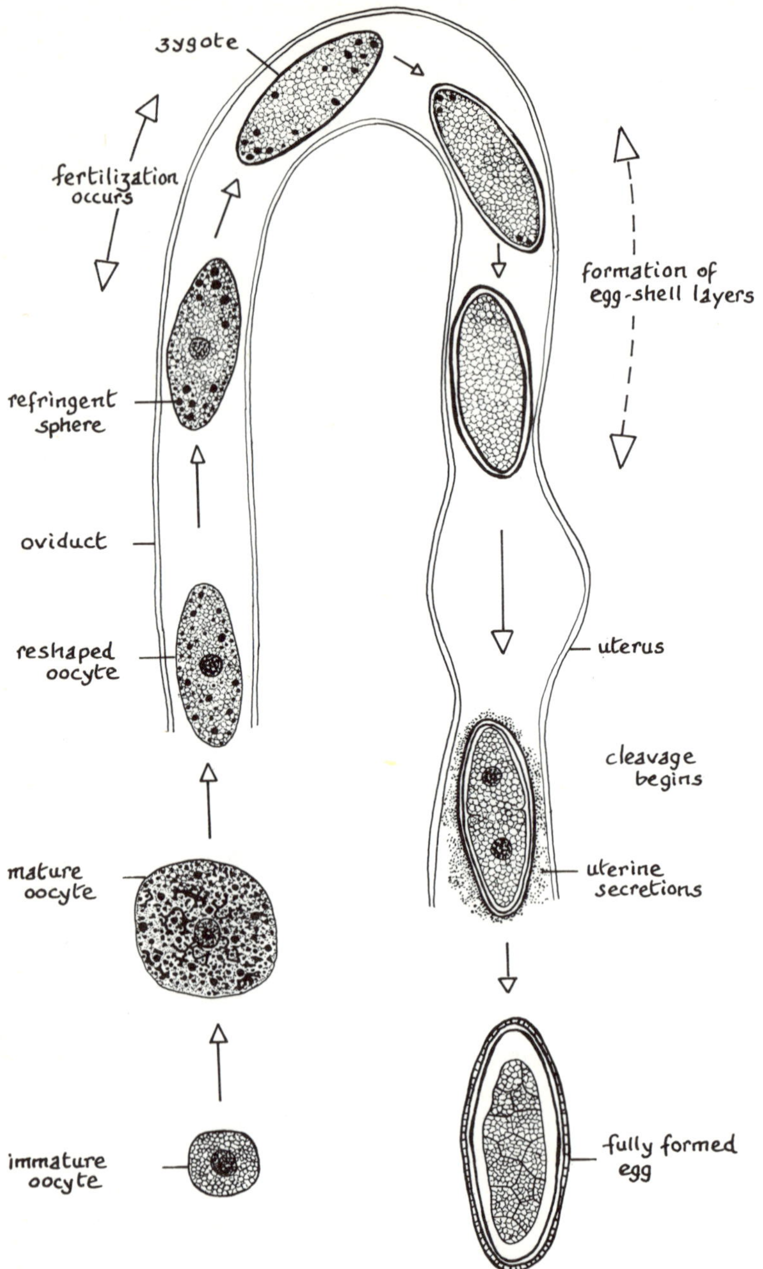


Fig. 7.30. Diagrammatic representation of eggshell formation in *Aspiculuris tetraptera* (Nematoda) (after Anya, 1964, *Parasitology*, **54**, 699).

development occurring as the egg arrives in the uterus (fig. 7.26). The development of the eggshell in nematodes occurs during the passage of the zygote along the reproductive tract. The events are illustrated diagrammatically for the mouse pinworm, *Aspiculuris tetraptera*, in fig. 7.30, and can be imagined for *Ascaris* by reference to fig. 7.25.

The nematode *Heterakis gallinarum* is the intermediate host of the protozoon *Histomonas meleagridis*, which causes enterohepatitis in domestic poultry. The nematode's eggs are the main agents of transmission of *Histomonas* between birds, and the mode of entry of *Histomonas* into the egg of *Heterakis* has only recently been discovered. The nematode lives in the caecal lumen of birds, where it ingests *Histomonas*. The protozoa develop for a time in the nematode's intestinal cells before breaking out into the body cavity and invading the reproductive tract. In female *Heterakis*, the *Histomonas* penetrate the mature oocytes before fertilization has occurred. Thus *Histomonas* benefits from the protection afforded by the resistant eggshell of *Heterakis*.

### 7.7.2. *Release of eggs*

Adult worms generally occupy a site which has an opening for the escape of eggs to the environment of the next host in the life cycle. Those worms which live in and around the alimentary tract or urinogenital system are provided with an obvious route for egg dispersal, and those in the respiratory tract have a connection with the alimentary route through the oesophagus. Parasitic worms in the cavities, tissues, blood and lymphatic system have become dependent on the feeding activities of vectors for transmission. However, *Coitocaecum anaspidis* sometimes reproduces as a result of progenesis involving the metacercarial stage in the body cavity of a freshwater shrimp. Eggs are laid within the metacercarial cyst and presumably do not reach the water until the shrimp has died and decomposed.

Some evidence indicates that the release of eggs may be rhythmical rather than continuous. Female *Enterobius vermicularis* emigrate from the large intestine to the perianal skin of man to deposit their eggs, particularly between 2100 hours and midnight. The rat pinworm, *Syphacia muris*, deposits most of its eggs when the host is quiescent during the daytime. The eggs of *A. tetraptera* are released intermittently rather than continuously and the release seems to be connected with the host's feeding activity. Similarly, gravid proglottides of the cestode *Davainea proglottina*, which inhabits the small intestine of chickens, are discharged mainly during the last few hours of daylight when the feeding activity of the host is minimal.

# 8. Aspects of development

The growth of an organism is the permanent increase in mass produced by the formation of more cytoplasm or the secretion of extracellular products. It is surprisingly difficult to measure. Since an increase in weight may arise from the accumulation of fluid rather than the production of new tissue, more reliable measures of growth may be obtained from estimations of dry weight and of nitrogen, protein and nucleic acid content. During early life, the process called differentiation produces many morphological changes, and a healthy organism becomes a complex unit of interdependent cells, tissues and organs. The development of an organism consists of growth and differentiation. During development, the parasitic stages of a worm incorporate energy and materials directly from the host. Consequently, the growth of a parasite is usually even more difficult to study and measure than that of a free-living organism. The investigator of a parasite's growth has to contend not only with the range of variation which characterizes any group of organisms of the same species, but also with the fact that hosts of the same species are also very variable in their own growth responses and in their suitability as hosts. When cockroaches of the same age, strain and sex are each given the same number of infective eggs of *Moniliformis* obtained from female worms of the same age and strain, parasites in several stages of development can usually be found in any one of the cockroaches until sufficient time has elapsed for every parasite to have reached the cystacanth stage (fig. 8.21).

The development of worms in intermediate hosts usually consists of the differentiation of all the organs and tissues, except for the gonads, together with relatively little growth, whereas development in definitive hosts usually consists of the differentiation of the gonads, maturation of the gametes and the growth of the somatic tissues. One feature of the development of worms is the rapid rate of differentiation of so many species. The tapeworm *Hymenolepis* completes its differentiation in the body cavity of *Tribolium* sp. in about 8 days if the beetles are kept at about 30 °C on a diet of enriched flour and raisins. Some tapeworms also grow to great lengths in their definitive hosts. *Diphyllobothrium latum* may reach a length of about 9 m after a few months. Clearly its rate of growth is rapid, but so is that of any metazoan animal which has also started from the fusion of two cells.

In many organisms, changes of size are usually accompanied by changes of shape and proportion. A free-living organism which is dependent on obtaining some substance by diffusion is constrained by this requirement to remain as a flattened creature with the maximum surface area that its bulk will permit. Marked changes of shape are observed during the development of digeneans, cestodes and acanthocephalans (figs. 8.3–8.21), and some authorities consider that metamorphosis occurs. Metamorphosis involves a change of form and structure during development. Clearly, by this definition, digenean development is metamorphic and nematode development is not, but the metamorphosis is not as complete as that which occurs in holometabolous insects. Sometimes the changes of shape are associated with some degree of growth and sometimes they are not. Changes of shape during development are of interest because they may result in the redeployment of cells, so that some will come into contact with each other for the first time, while others will lose contact. Similarly, some cells will lose or gain contact with the external environment. Imagine the redistribution of cells that will occur if an organism changes from a spherical to a flattened shape without any major increase in the number of its cells.

## 8.1. *Monogenea*

Monogenean development consists of growth and the gradual acquisition of adult characters by the larval stages once the oncomiracidium has settled on the appropriate host. In the case of *Diclidophora denticulata*, which inhabits the gills of *Gadus virens*, the ciliated coat of the oncomiracidium is discarded. The form of the haptor changes from one bearing paired hooks to one having paired clamps (figs. 8.1, 8.2). A considerable amount of growth occurs, the geminal primordia appear and the alimentary tract develops. As with all parasites developing on or in poikilothermic hosts, the rate of development varies with temperature.

Although the general pattern of morphological changes occurring during development may be similar for different species of monogenean fluke, there are more striking behavioural and physiological differences between species. The life cycle of *Polystoma* is apparently synchronized with the sexual maturation of its frog host. The flukes, which live in the frogs' bladders, attain maturity and lay eggs as the frogs enter water and begin their breeding cycles, and the oncomiracidia hatch in time to invade the gills of the tadpoles. When the tadpoles begin to change into frogs, the juvenile flukes leave the gills, scramble over the bellies of their hosts and enter the bladder by way of the cloaca.

## 8.2. *Digenea*

Several features of digenean development are illustrated in figs. 8.3–8.7, which refer to the liver fluke, *Fasciola*. As soon as the miracidium has penetrated a suitable snail, the ciliated coat is lost and

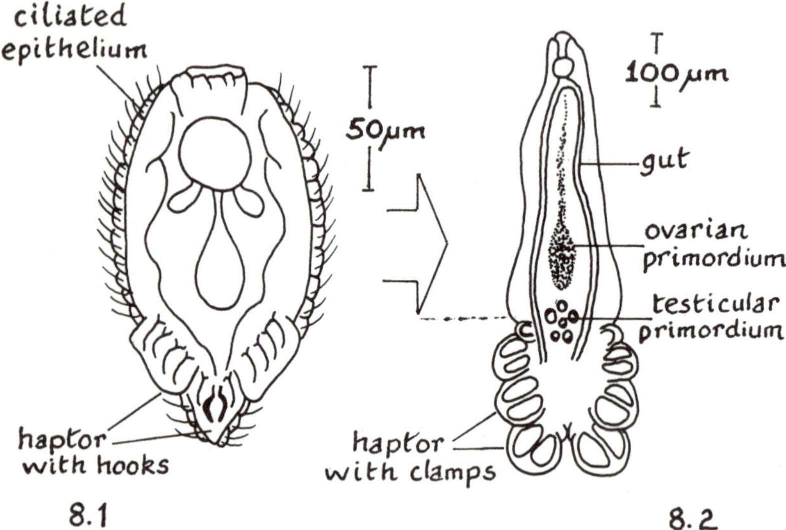


Figs. 8.1 and 8.2. Morphological changes during the development of *Diclidophora denticulata* (Monogenea) (after Frankland, 1955, *Parasitology*, **45**, 313). 8.1. Young larva. 8.2. Advanced larva.

the young sporocyst, as the organism is now known, changes shape by rounding up. The sporocyst then increases in size, largely by growth and multiplication of the balls of germinal cells which are confined within its thin tegument (fig. 8.5). A sporocyst has no gut, nutrients being absorbed through the tegument. Some evidence suggests that sporocysts may release lytic substances which help to provide a supply of absorbable material from the tissues of the host. In time, the sporocysts give rise to the more complex rediae† (fig. 8.6), which

† The redia is named after the Italian scientist Franciso Redi (1626–1697).

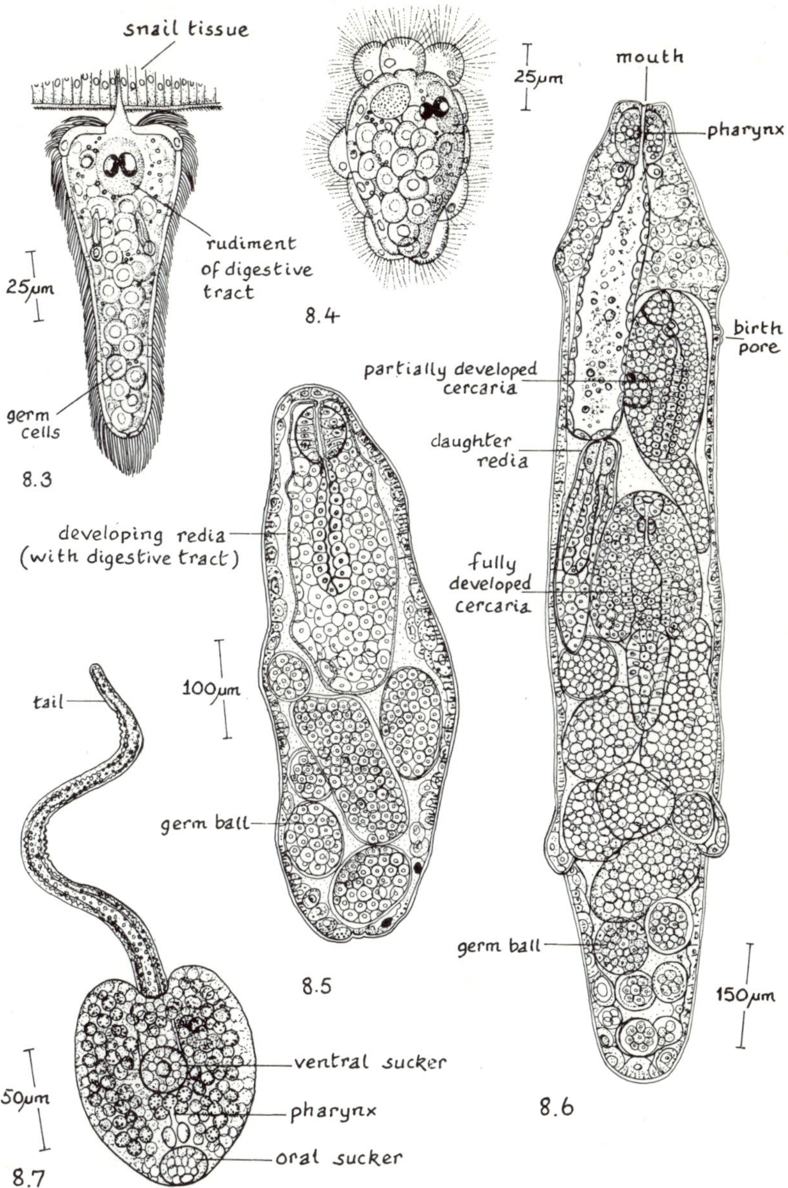


Figs. 8.3–8.7. Aspects of the development of *Fasciola hepatica* (Digenea) (after Thomas, 1883). 8.3. Miracidium engaged in boring into the snail intermediate host. 8.4. A young parasite recently arrived in the tissues of the snail. 8.5. A sporocyst with a redia at its upper end. 8.6. A redia containing a daughter redia and cercariae. 8.7. A fully developed cercaria.

possess a gut and ingest the cells of their hosts. These, in turn, give rise to more rediae and to cercariae (fig. 8.7). Most of the development of *Fasciola* in the snail, and of other species of digenean fluke in their snail hosts, takes place in the snail's digestive gland.

In some digeneans, sporocysts and rediae are difficult to distinguish, and in *Fasciola* the environmental temperature of the snail can influence whether daughter rediae are produced or not. Some workers prefer to use the term 'germinal sacs' to include such stages as mother and daughter sporocysts, mother and daughter rediae and other digenean developmental stages which contribute to the production of cercariae. All the cercariae formed as the result of one miracidium becoming established in a snail and giving rise to germinal sacs are believed to have the same genome. They arise by polyembryony from the original zygote which gave rise to the miracidium. It is thought that the first mitotic cleavage of the zygote produces two unequal cells. One cell leads to the development of the body of the miracidum, while the other gives rise to the germinal cells. This functional segregation of the cell lines continues throughout the sporocysts and rediae in which the germinal cells are organized into balls (figs. 8.5, 8.6). All the cells of the germinal line are assumed to divide mitotically so that true asexual reproduction occurs without any loss of chromosomes. In some studies, a single miracidium of *Fasciola* has been found to give rise to about 600 cercariae, which first begin to escape from the snail about 5 weeks after the penetration of the miracidium. *Fasciola* is fortunate in that its common snail host, *Lymnaea truncatula*, also has a prodigious reproductive rate when optimum conditions prevail. A single *L. truncatula* has the reproductive potential to start a population which could reach about 160 000 within 3 months.

## 8.3. *Cestoda*

The development of tapeworms follows the general pattern shown in fig. 8.8. The oncospheres always emigrate to a site in the body tissues of the intermediate host irrespective of whether it is an invertebrate or a vertebrate. Metamorphosis occurs and the larval stages are often referred to as metacestodes. The term cestode is usually reserved for a tapeworm in its definitive host where the proglottides are found. The process of proglottis formation is not fully understood. Small proglottides develop in the neck region just behind the scolex, and as their growth occurs they are displaced caudally along the strobila. The development of *Hymenolepis* (figs. 8.9–8.15) is relatively simple, since there is no asexual budding of the type that occurs during the

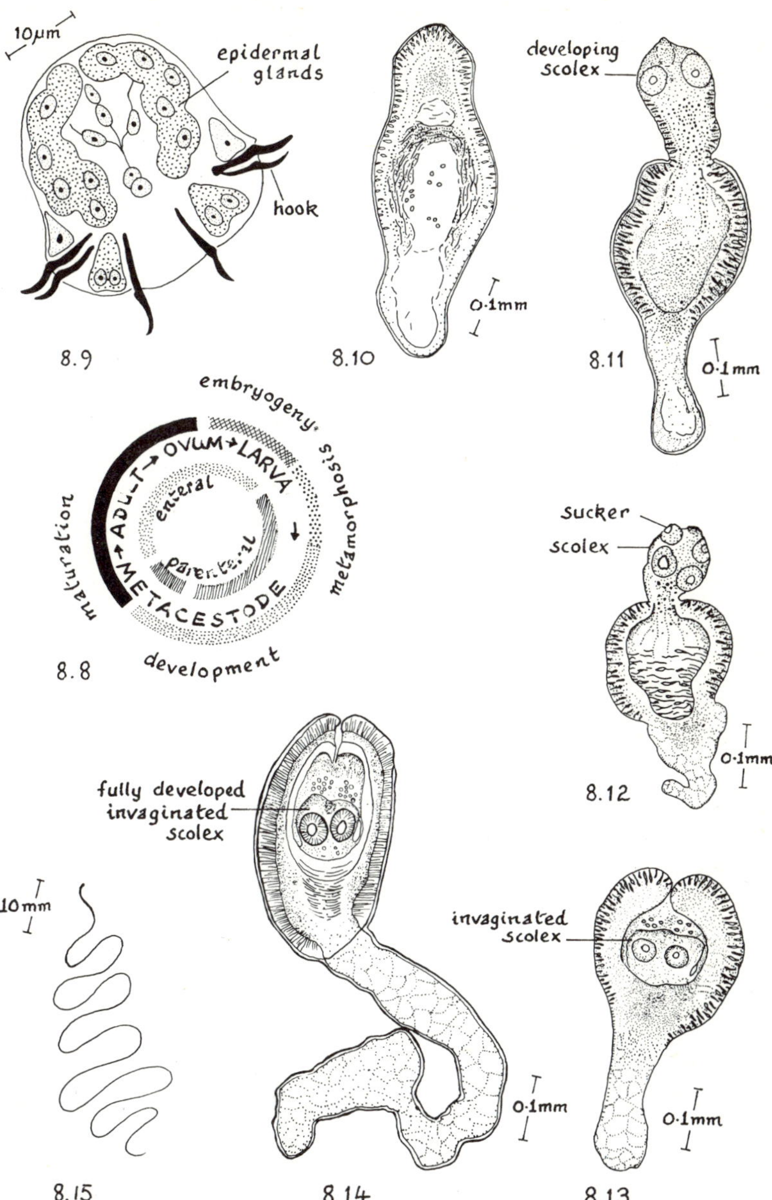


Figs. 8.8–8.15. Aspects of the development of cestodes. 8.8. The basic developmental pattern (after Freeman, 1973, *Adv. Parasit.*, **11**, 481). 8.9–8.15. Stages in the development of *Hymenolepis* spp. from oncosphere (8.9) to adult (8.15) (after Voge and Heyneman, 1957, *Univ. Cal. Publ. Zool.*, **59**, 549; Smyth, 1969, *The Physiology of Cestodes*).

development of *Paricterotaenia paradoxa* in earthworms and *Echinococcus granulosus* in sheep (see fig. 3.35).

Development in poikilothermic hosts is retarded when the temperature falls and is accelerated when the temperature rises. If the temperature rises above certain limits, abnormal development of the metacestode may occur. When mealworms infected with *Hymenolepis* were kept at a temperature of 38.5 or 40 °C for 24 hours, during the period when maximum growth of the parasite is expected to occur, the scoleces (fig. 8.14) were not withdrawn and the cysticercoids were not infective to rats. The mealworms withstand such periods of elevated temperature without any obvious ill effects.

## 8.4. *Acanthocephala*

Acanthocephalan development (figs. 8.16–8.21) is less varied than that of digeneans and cestodes. The acanthor larva contains a central mass of nuclei from which the different primordia of the various organ systems arise once the parasite has reached the haemocoele of its intermediate host. The acanthor does not possess a body cavity, but this is formed together with most of the organs during the acanthella stages (fig. 8.19). *Moniliformis* is an archiacanthocephalan (table 1.1) and its proboscis develops in an everted position before being withdrawn on the formation of the cystacanth (fig. 8.21). Palaeacanthocephalans and eoacanthocephalans are different in that development of the proboscis begins with the tissue inverted. As development proceeds, the proboscis tissue is everted, only to be withdrawn once the cystacanth stage is reached.

## 8.5. *Nematoda*

The development of nematodes shows no metamorphosis and there occurs a steady change from juvenile to adult stage irrespective of whether intermediate hosts are involved or not. The cell number of most somatic tissues of a nematode is believed to be constant, growth involving an increase in cell size instead of cell number. Growth is interrupted at regular intervals when moulting takes place. A representation of the growth curve of a hypothetical nematode is shown in fig. 8.22. Four moults occur and it is now recognized that growth may be continuous throughout the moults, or growth may be arrested just before, during and after a moult. There is no satisfactory explanation of the biological reason for this moulting. In insects, the exoskeleton becomes tanned and inextensible, and must be shed if the animal is to increase in size. The period immediately after moulting, but before the cuticle has become hardened, is the period when insects expand their bodies and accommodate their increased bulk more comfortably. In some nematodes, however, the cuticle continues to grow in thickness after the final moult.

Moulting in nematodes may be considered as a four-stage process. First, some stimulus is received and neurosecretory material is discharged from the nervous system. Secondly, the old cuticle becomes separated. Thirdly, the new cuticle is secreted by the hypodermis while portions of the old cuticle may or may not be reabsorbed into the hypodermis. Most of the old cuticle is reabsorbed

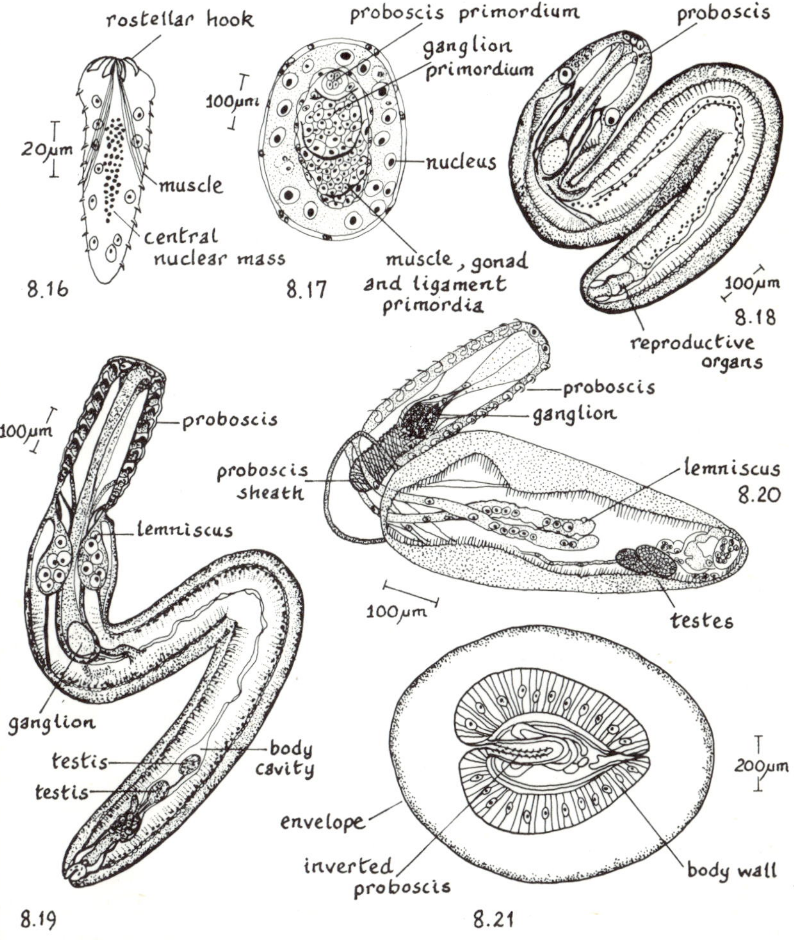


Figs. 8.16–8.21. Aspects of the development of *Moniliformis dubius* (Acanthocephala) (after King and Robinson, 1967, *J. Parasit.*, **53**, 142; Nicholas, 1967, *Adv. Parasit.*, **5**, 205). 8.16. Acanthor. 8.17–8.20. Acanthella stages. 8.21. Cystacanth.

when a developing nematode moults within the confines of an egg. Larvae of *Ascaris* moult once within their eggs, while those of *Nematodirus battus* moult twice. Fourthly, the old cuticle is shed. During moulting, the cuticular linings of the buccal cavity, pharynx, excretory pore and rectal region are shed as well as the outer covering of the body.

The third-stage larvae of many nematodes are infective if swallowed (Chapter 3). Such larvae are often encased in the cuticle which separated from the second-stage larvae during the second moult. The process whereby the third-stage larva escapes from the old, detached,

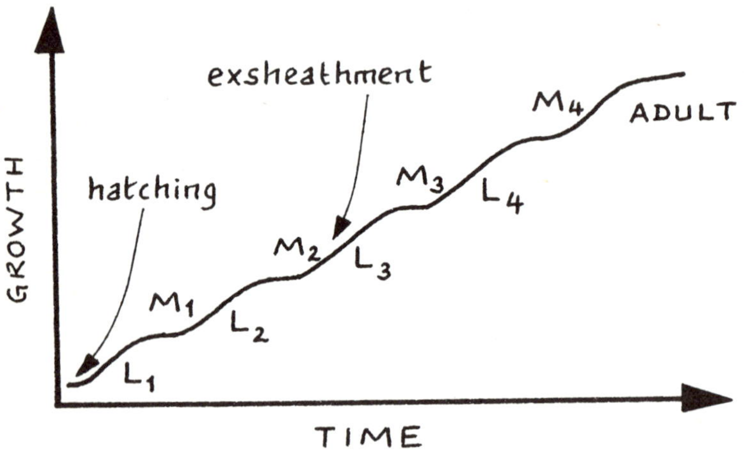


Fig. 8.22. A hypothetical growth curve of an animal parasitic nematode (after Lee, 1965).

cuticle is called exsheathment (fig. 8.22) and it represents the completion of the second moult. Exsheathment appears to be initiated by a stimulus which prompts the release of exsheathing fluid from the excretory pore. In *Haemonchus contortus*, the high concentrations of environmental carbon dioxide or carbonic acid, which are found in the rumen of sheep, may contribute to the exsheathing stimulus. Exsheathing fluid, which attacks the sheath in a preformed region near the excretory pore, may be a solution of proteolytic enzymes. *Dictyocaulus viviparus* is a nematode which lives in the lungs of cattle. The third-stage larvae of this species also enter their hosts by the oral route in an ensheathed state. Exsheathment occurs posterior to the rumen, and it appears that pepsin contributes to the exsheathing stimulus of *Dictyocaulus*.

## 8.6. *Longevity*

Many factors may be assumed to affect the life-span of parasitic worms. Some estimations of the maximum life-spans of adults are given in table 8.1. These values have been obtained from investigations in which care was taken to avoid the establishment of subsequent infections. In this type of study, there is always the chance that larval stages might survive in an arrested state and later replace the adult worms which had died.

TABLE 8.1. *Some observations on the ages attained by parasitic worms in definitive hosts. (Remember that many features of parasitism affect the life expectancy of parasites.)*

| | |
|---|---|
| MONOGENEA | ACANTHOCEPHALA |
| *Polystoma integerrimum* 6 years (frog) | *Moniliformis dubius* 5 months (rat) |
| DIGENEA | NEMATODA |
| *Fasciola hepatica* 11 years (sheep) | *Ascaris lumbricoides* 1 year (man) |
| *Schistosoma mansoni* 19 years (man) | *Dirofilaria immitis* 5 years (dog) |
| | *Enterobius vermicularis* 8 weeks (man) |
| CESTODA | Hookworm 7 years (man) |
| *Hymenolepis diminuta* life of host (rat) | *Nippostrongylus brasiliensis* 2 weeks (rat) |
| *Moniezia expansa* 10 weeks (sheep) | |
| *Taenia saginata* 13 years (man) | *Wuchereria bancrofti* 17 years (man) |

The immune response of the host is an important influence in the longevity of worms. The nematode *Nippostrongylus* elicits a strong protective immune response in rats with the result that most worms from a primary infection are expelled from the small intestine after about 14 days (9.2.2). During the first week of a primary infection, however, the rat's immune responses have not yet been activated against the *Nippostrongylus*, and young adult worms may be transplanted by surgical techniques from one rat to another, provided that the recipient has had no previous infection with *Nippostrongylus*. Presumably this trick of removing the worms ahead of the immune response could be repeated time and again, enabling an estimate of the potential life-span to be made. *Nippostrongylus* might also survive for a long time in an immuno-suppressed host, although immuno-suppressed animals can be difficult to keep alive unless special germ-free facilities are available for their care. One series of transplantation experiments was made with *Hymenolepis*, in which tapeworms from the same original population were kept alive for 14 years. The scoleces and parts of the neck region were transplanted from one group of rats to another on each occasion and the remainder of the strobilae were discarded. Since the longevity of the worms greatly exceeded that of the rats, it is possible to speculate that the scolex and anterior part of the neck of *Hymenolepis* do not age in the same manner as the rest of the worm. The life-span of *Hymenolepis* in a rat may extend until the death of the rat.

## 8.7. *Cultivation* in vitro

Our knowledge of the development, nutrition and metabolism of many parasitic worms will remain superficial until the worms can be maintained and grown *in vitro* by methods similar to those used in tissue culture. Elimination of the host might lead to a loss of stimuli for the parasite and a totally different environment, but controlled experiments would be possible, vaccines might be produced, and fewer animals would be required to act as experimental hosts in laboratories.

Ideally, growth and development *in vitro* should follow the same pattern and time course as *in vivo*. One of the major problems is deciding which parameters should be studied to indicate whether growth *in vitro* is proceeding satisfactorily. Another problem arises from the fact that many worms spend a relatively long time in growing to full size. Consequently, the apparatus and culture medium must be kept sterile for an equivalent period. Microbiologists may not need to maintain their cultures free from contamination for more than a few days, whereas the parasitologist may need sterile conditions for his worm for a few weeks. Curiously enough, several of the worms which have been kept in culture for a reasonable period normally live in close association with bacteria in the alimentary tract. Nevertheless failure to maintain sterile conditions *in vitro* would soon have led to another disappointing experiment.

*Hymenolepis* was the first parasitic worm to be grown *in vitro*. Cysticercoids of *Hymenolepis* were activated *in vitro* (see table 3.2) and were introduced on to a substratum of filter paper in a special sterile apparatus. Presumably the filter paper simulated in some manner contact between the worm and the mucosa of the host's small intestine. The nutrient medium flowed continuously over the worms and so removed excretory products and perhaps reproduced other physical aspects of the intestinal environment. The worms *in vitro* matured in 15 days and their proglottides could not be distinguished from those of worms of the same stage of development from rats.

# 9. Host resistance and allergic reactivity to parasitic worms

At the beginning of this book, parasitism was presented as a delicate physiological equilibrium between the activity of the parasite and the resistance of the host. Some concepts of the extent of the forms of host resistance and the variety of the terminology are set out in fig. 9.1. Resistance can be classified according to whether it is non-specific or specific in character. In general, non-specific responses to infection are those with which an animal is endowed at birth, whereas specific responses develop actively as an animal ages and acquires greater experience of foreign organisms and intruders. The terms which are used to describe different host responses tend to reflect the interpretation given by an investigator to his observations on a particular form of response. Use of the word 'immune' ought to mean that a host is now exempt from contagion or is well protected from the parasite in question. This is not always the case, and, although some hosts do mount immune responses which actually expel the parasite or curb its activities, other hosts respond in a way which may cause further damage to themselves. Many workers now think of specific anti-parasite responses as allergic reactions. Adoption of the word 'allergic' is to be recommended because it does not imply anything except that a host is responding to the presence of materials that are recognized as 'not-self'.

Parasitologists often refer to the susceptibility of a host to a particular parasite. Various features of the biology of the host may reduce its susceptibility to infection by a parasitic worm or even render it insusceptible under natural conditions without any participation from the non-specific and specific mechanisms of resistance. For example, the structure and integrity of tissue barriers like the skin of mammals or the exoskeleton of arthropods may prevent the penetration of parasites; conditions in the alimentary tract of one animal may not promote the growth of the parasites of another and *vice versa*; the natural diet and feeding behaviour of an animal may ensure that it never ingests the infective stages of a worm which would be able to thrive in its tissues; and so on. One aim of modern health education in tropical countries is to stimulate communities to alter aspects of their behaviour and so become less susceptible to parasitic infection. This approach may eventually prove to be the cheapest and most effective form of control of parasitic disease. Climatic and other ecological factors in the environment of a host and the infective stages of its parasites also contribute to susceptibility to infection. It is important that the non-specific and specific responses made by hosts against parasites (fig. 9.1) are not confused with the other factors which have a major bearing on susceptibility. In all cases, however, the physiological and nutritional status of the host may well influence the outcome of a host–parasite relationship.

Before turning to survey the resistance of hosts to parasitic worms, it is worth reflecting that in certain cases successful host resistance may be as important for the survival of a parasitic species as it is for the host species. If all hosts died as a result of a specific parasitic onslaught, the parasites would become extinct for want of an environment. It is also stressed that the following survey of mechanisms of host resistance and allergic reactivity is bound to be brief and incomplete within the context of a short book on one branch of parasitology.

## 9.1. *Non-specific responses*

### 9.1.1. *Invertebrate hosts* (fig. 9.1)

The evidence strongly suggests that the major resistance of coelenterates, annelids, molluscs, arthropods and echinoderms is provided by cells suspended in their body fluids. Metchnikoff, towards the end of the 19th century, observed cells surrounding thorns which he had pushed into the body cavities of starfish larvae, and later he saw cells engulfing fungal spores which he had injected into *Daphnia*. He coined the name phagocytes for these defence cells and, although phagocytes are nowadays much better known in vertebrates, there is little doubt that phagocytosis is the major means whereby invading micro-organisms are neutralized in the bodies of invertebrates.

Worms and other parasites are too large to be engulfed by a phagocytic cell. Most work on the resistance of invertebrates to metazoan parasites has been carried out on insects. An effective defence reaction, which is known to occur in at least 14 orders of insect, is made by the blood cells or haemocytes and is called encapsulation. Haemocytes adhere to the foreign body and flatten themselves over its surface in a reaction very different from their

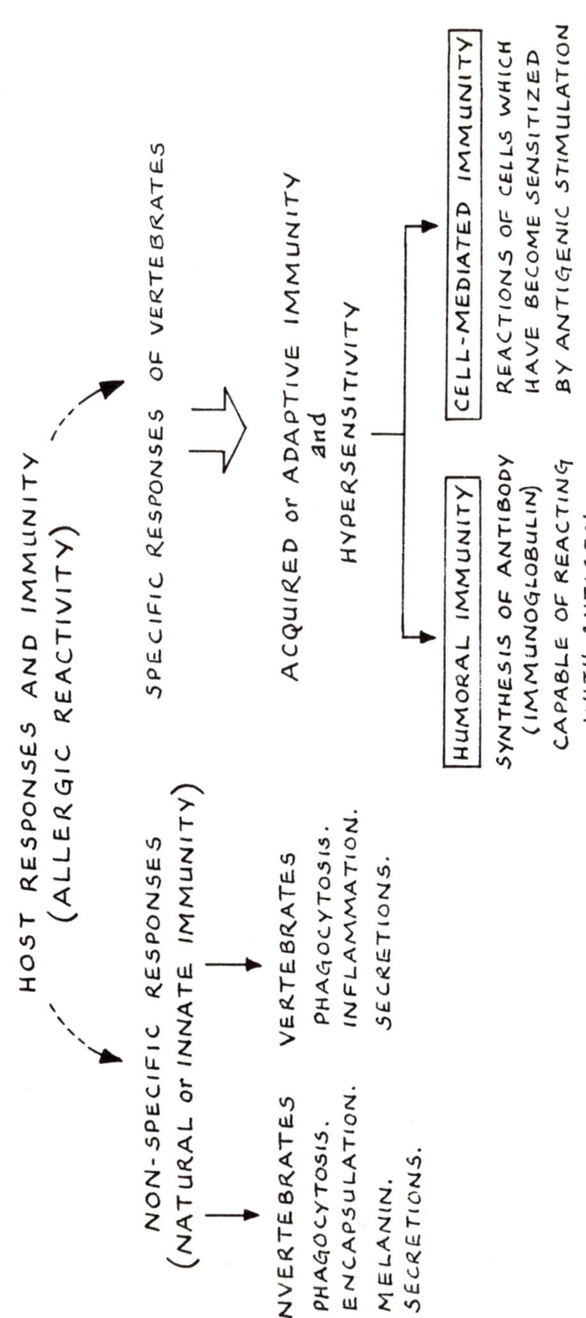


Fig. 9.1. A simplified scheme of host responses.

response to their own healthy tissues. The mass of haemocytes increases until a particular size has been attained. In some cases, living objects may deprived of nutrients and oxygen and so be killed by the capsule of haemocytes. Capsules begin to assemble as soon as the foreign body intrudes into tissues or cavities in which the haemocytes are to be found (fig. 9.2). After some time, the capsules shrink and connective tissue is formed in and amongst the layers of cells. The dark, inert pigment melanin is not infrequently associated with the cellular reaction against a foreign organism; its formation is thought to involve the participation of the blood cells. The developmental stage, physiological state and blood-cell count of the species of insect are some of the factors which affect encapsulation.

Two examples will serve to show how encapsulation works in practice against developing parasitic worms in insects. Eggs of *Dipylidium caninum*, a common tapeworm of cats and dogs, are ingested by the larvae of cat fleas. The oncospheres emerge from the eggs and bore through the intestinal wall into the body cavity, where they are exposed to the haemocytes. Some of the developing tapeworms are completely encapsulated and destroyed (fig. 9.3), but those parasites which survive until the prepupal stage in the flea's development, when encapsulation is retarded, are able to grow rapidly. Acanthors of *Moniliformis* (fig. 8.16) are also often encapsulated when they reach the body cavity of the cockroach *Periplaneta americana*. After a few days, the encapsulating cells are observed to be present but no longer making close contact with the surface of the acanthor. One interpretation of electron micrographs prepared at this point in the development of *Moniliformis* is that the parasite produces at its surface membranous material which repels the haemocytes (fig. 9.4). The parasite's development is completed within a jacket of membranous material which may include some haemocytes and their fragmented remains. Not all the acanthors of *Moniliformis* are successful in their development. For a known dose of eggs given to a cockroach, some eggs fail to hatch in the gut, some acanthors fail to enter the body cavity and some are vanquished by the host's defence reaction.

Thus we have seen that the relationships evolved between parasitic worms and insects enable some individuals to complete development despite the attention of the haemocytes. Other parasitic worms, for example *Hymenolepis*, complete their development in the body cavities of flour beetles without seeming to stimulate the encapsulating response. The ability of a flour beetle, however, to react by encapsulation can be demonstrated experimentally by injecting other

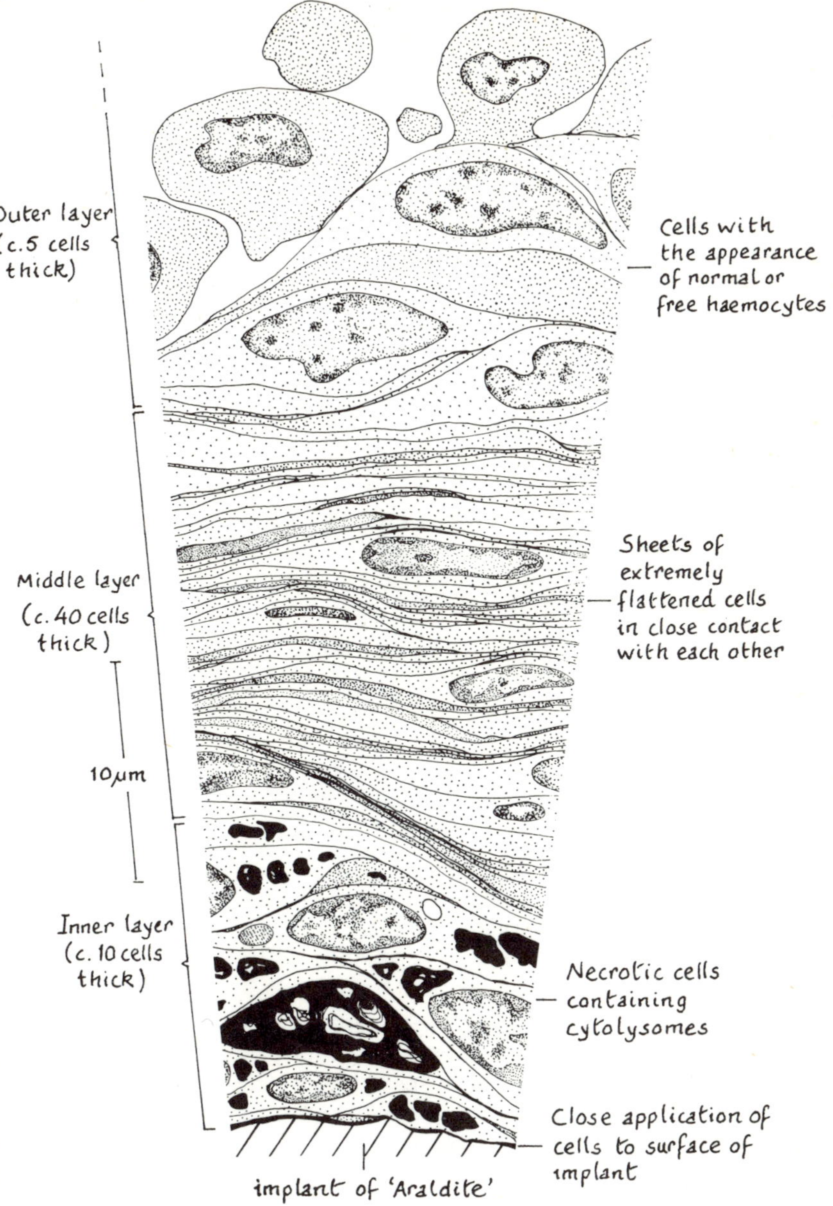


Fig. 9.2. Diagrammatic reconstruction, based on electron micrographs, of a section through a capsule of haemocytes 72 h after a small implant of 'Araldite' had been placed in the body cavity of a caterpillar of the flour moth, *Ephestia kuehniella* (after Grimstone, Rotheram and Salt, 1967).

foreign bodies directly into the body cavity. In addition to *Hymenolepis*, the normal healthy tissues of the flour beetle do not stimulate encapsulation either. The fundamental question to be answered with regard to the defence reactions of insects is how do the haemocytes distinguish between self and not-self? Clearly the developing stages of *Hymenolepis* are foreign to the insect, but either they are not recognized as such or other mechanisms act to circumvent the haemocytic response. Possible mechanisms might include (*a*) suppression of the cellular response by secretions of the parasite, (*b*) rapid destruction of the capsule by secretions of the parasite (*c*) the

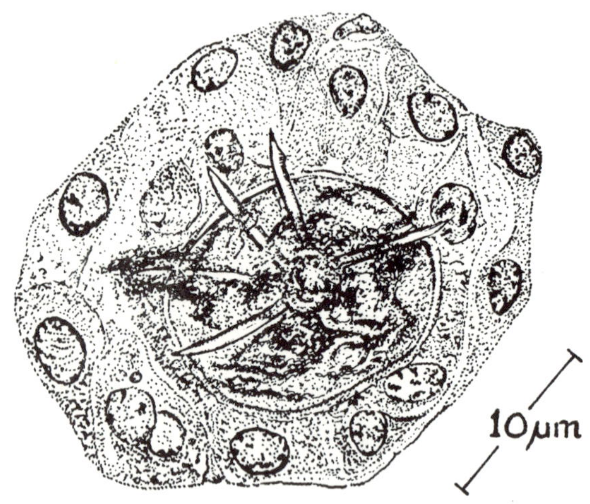


Fig. 9.3. A capsule formed by haemocytes of the cat flea, *Ctenocephalides felis*, around a developmental stage of *Dipylidium caninum* (Cestoda). Pigment and remains of the parasite can be seen (after Salt, 1963, *Parasitology*, **53**, 527).

acquisition by the parasite of a camouflaged surface by means of adsorbed molecules from the host's body fluids, and (*d*) the possession by the parasite of a surface inherently similar to that of the internal surfaces of the host. This topic is worthy of much thought and research, not only because it presents an intellectual challenge but also because it is directly involved in the choice of agents for the biological control of injurious insects.

### 9.1.2. *Vertebrate hosts* (fig. 9.1)

The healthy vertebrate body appears to be remarkably efficient at removing microbes and certain particles from internal circulation. This function is carried out by phagocytic cells, of which the two main types in mammals are the polymorphonuclear leukocytes and the macrophages (figs. 9.5, 9.6). Phagocytosis may not be very important as a direct line of defence for the vertebrate host against relatively large parasitic worms. Its main contribution during helminth infections will probably be the engulfment of the bacteria which enter the tissues through the lesions caused by the activities of worms. Some micro-organisms, however, are not destroyed by phagocytes but flourish within them. A consideration of phagocytosis illustrates the

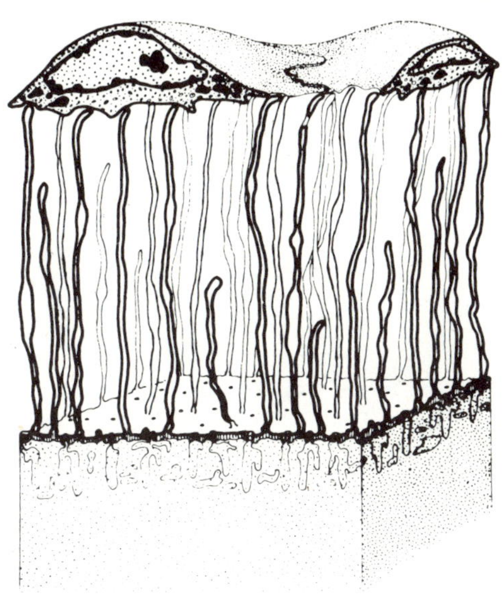

Fig. 9.4. Diagrammatic interpretation, based on electron micrographs, to show how membranous material produced from the surface of an acanthor of *Moniliformis dubius* (Acanthocephala) might repel the host's haemocytes (after Crompton, 1975, *Symp. Soc. Exp. Biol.*, **29**, 467).

difficulties which arise when host responses are classified as either non-specific or specific (fig. 9.1). In mammals, the phagocytosis of a particular agent is often enhanced by the presence of opsonins, which are antibodies found in the serum of subjects immunized against the agent. Other circumstances are known in which non-specific and specific responses act in collaboration rather than independently.

Vertebrates often react against parasitic worms by an inflammatory response. When a foreign object arrives in the tissues, localized swelling occurs as a result of the dilation of the blood capillaries in the region, and then leukocytes and fibroblasts accumulate at the site and the object is surrounded by cells in a manner not unlike encapsulation

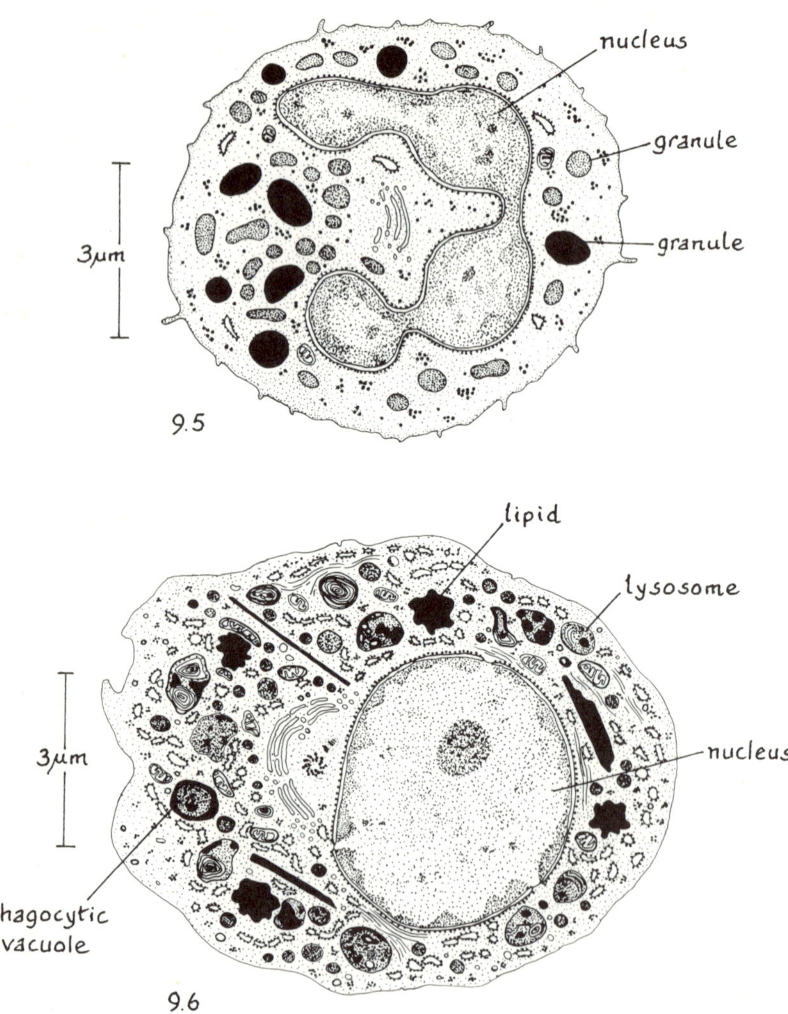


Figs. 9.5 and 9.6. Interpretations based on electron micrographs, of the structure of mammalian leukocytes (after Lentz, 1971, *Cell Fine Structure*). 9.5. Polymorphonuclear leukocyte. These phagocytic cells comprise about half the leukocytes in the blood. They are active in the early stages of inflammation. 9.6. Macrophage. These cells are often phagocytic and play an important co-operative role with lymphocytes in specific responses.

in insects. Eventually the object is enclosed in connective tissue, and calcification may occur, as in the case of long-standing infections of *Trichinella spiralis* (fig. 3.43).

## 9.2. *Specific responses of vertebrates* (fig. 9.1)

Although about 42 000 species of vertebrate are known to inhabit the earth, relatively few have been studied by immunologists. For the present, we must assume the general applicability of the extensive body of knowledge which has been obtained mainly from experiments on chickens, rats, mice, guinea-pigs and rabbits.

### 9.2.1. *Cellular basis of acquired immunity*

In birds and mammals, the cells involved in immune responses and allergic reactivity originate from stem cells in the bone marrow. The stem cells give rise to various cell types including small lymphocytes (fig. 9.7), which at a certain stage in the life of the animal become organized into two functionally distinct populations. Cells of one population are called T-cells, because they originate from lymphocytes which have been processed in some manner by the thymus gland, while those of the other population are called B-cells, because their ancestors are known to have been processed in the bursa of Fabricius if they are from birds or in some equivalent tissue in mammals. The lymph nodes and other organs of the body have an important role in providing centres for the activities of T and B-cells. In general, the B-cells are responsible for humoral antibody production, while the T-cells are responsible for cell-mediated immunity (fig. 9.1). Humoral responses involve the release of free antibodies, in the form of immunoglobulins, into the blood and body fluids. Cell-mediated responses are thought to depend mainly on cells which are said to be ‘sensitized’, which indicates that the cell surfaces are receptive in some way to antigens. Sensitized cells do not appear to produce antibody.

Higher vertebrates respond to a great variety of antigens by the production of an equally diverse range of antibodies; the secondary and subsequent responses to a given antigen are usually more rapid and powerful than the primary response. The reduced interval before the onset of the secondary response is strong evidence of the existence of some form of memory. Cell-mediated reponses are also specific and involve a memory in the healthy immuno-competent bird or mammal. These findings, together with the demonstration that specific receptor sites for antigen molecules are present at the surface

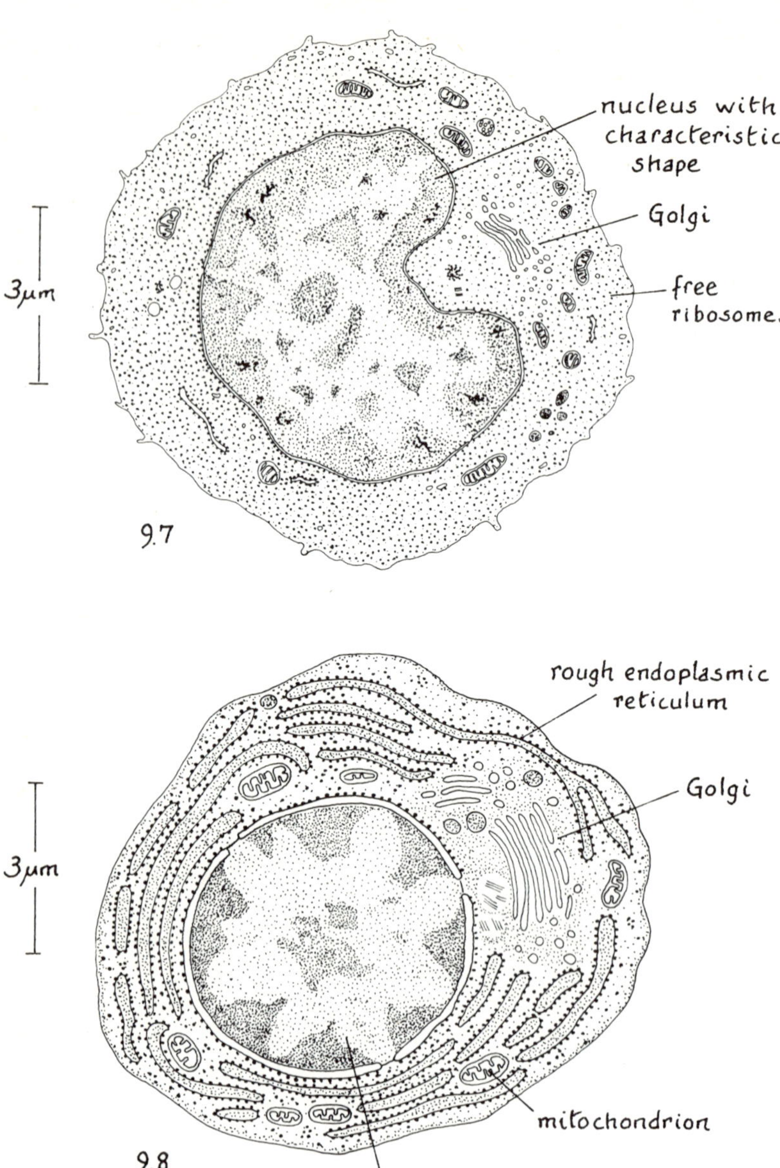


Figs. 9.7 and 9.8. Interpretations, based on electron micrographs, of the structure of mammalian leukocytes (after Lentz, 1971, *Cell Fine Structure*). 9.7. Small lymphocyte. These undifferentiated cells comprise about a quarter of the leukocytes in the blood. They are also found in various organs and tissues including the lymph, spleen, tonsils, intestinal wall, thymus and lymph nodes. 9.8. Plasma cell or transformed B-cell (fig. 9.9). These cells synthesize antibody.

of lymphocytes, have led to the development of the clonal selection theory to explain how immune and allergic responses occur.

A diagrammatic representation of the theory is set out in fig. 9.9. At present, the experimental evidence in support of the theory is more convincing for the functioning of the B-cells than of the T-cells. Antigen of a certain type binds to the B-cell with the appropriate receptor site. This contact then stimulates the proliferation of this cell to form a clone (fig. 9.9). Members of this clone transform into plasma cells (fig. 9.8) which synthesize and secrete antibody. Some members of the clone become memory cells which survive in the body

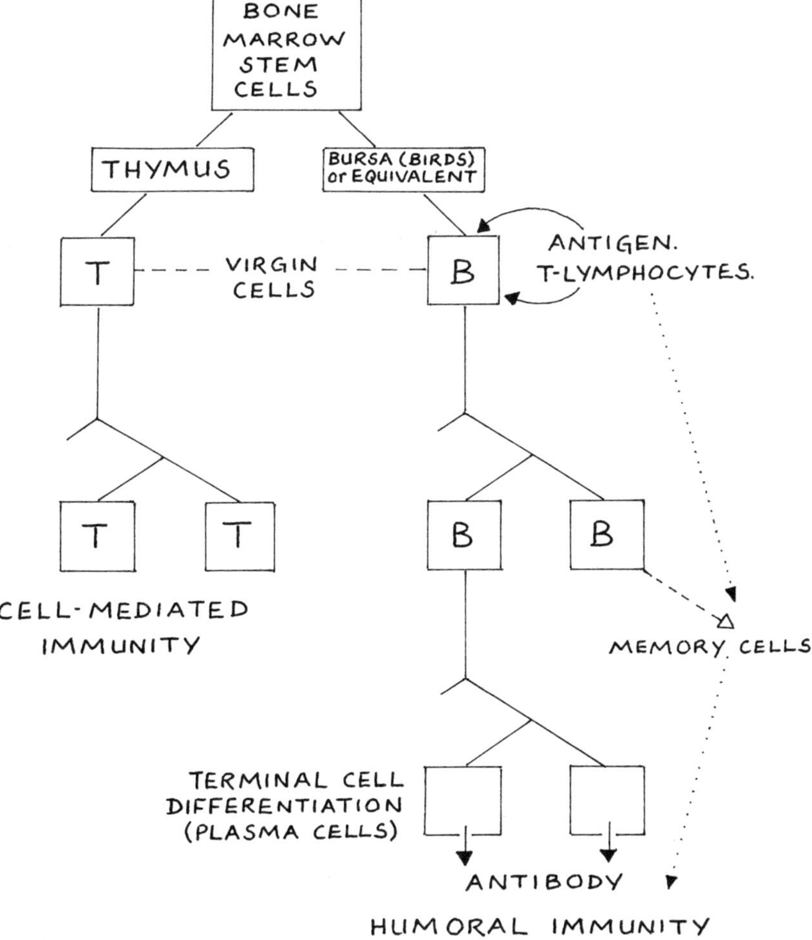


Fig. 9.9. A simplified scheme for the clonal selection theory (after Williamson, 1972).

with their specific receptors primed for the antigen. T-cells are also able to form clones, but less is known about this process. In fact, humoral responses appear to require the co-operation of both types of lymphocyte.

Finally, it must be stressed that the evolution of the immune or allergic process has provided higher animals with a most sensitive means of discriminating between self and not-self. The parallel evolution of mechanisms which allow parasitic worms to survive in hosts which are endowed with this discriminatory ability is one of the most fascinating aspects of biology.

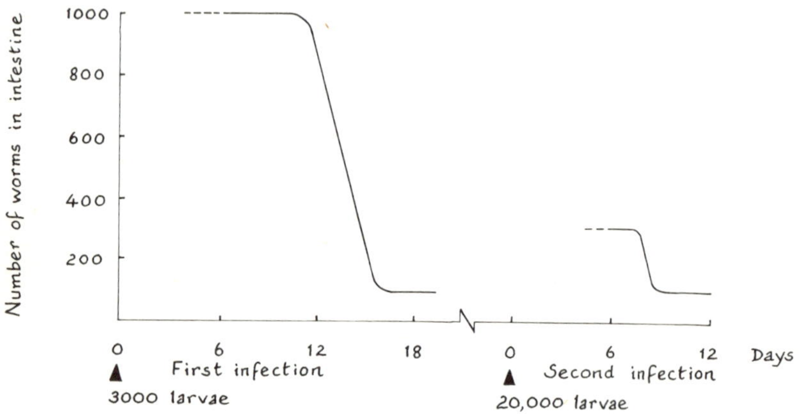


Fig. 9.10. The course of infection of *Nippostrongylus brasiliensis* (Nematoda) in rats showing the evidence which indicates that immunity develops.

### 9.2.2. *Responses against parasitic worms*

Although a large number of species of parasitic worm are of medical, agricultural and economic importance, few studies have been made to elucidate the nature of the immune and allergic responses which they evoke. Recently, however, progress has been made towards understanding how the rat responds to the presence of *Nippostrongylus*. The life cycle of this nematode (figs. 2.5, 4.5, 9.10) indicates that the population of adult worms becomes established in the anterior half of the small intestine of rats, of about 2 months of age or older, after a few days. During a first course of infection, egg production begins after about 5 days and continues for 7 or 8 days. Then it declines dramatically and most of the worms are lost (fig. 9.10). If rats in this condition are given a challenge infection of many more larvae than were used the first time, only a few worms reach the small intestine, they live for a shorter time, and few eggs are released (fig. 9.10). The relationship appears to involve the typical primary and secondary responses of an immuno-competent mammal to antigen. The rat retains the protective effect of its earlier experience of *Nippostrongylus* for some time. The antigen is associated principally with adult worms. Transplantation experiments have established that as few as ten adults can elicit protection, whereas larval stages stimulate little or no immunity to re-infection. The larval stages, however, are affected by the host response when it occurs.

Evidence for the participation of immune responses during the course of infection of *Nippostrongylus* has been obtained from several experimental approaches. First, a population of *Nippostrongylus* remains stable and is long-lived in an adult rat from which the thymus gland has been removed soon after birth. Secondly, the life span of the worm is prolonged if the rat is treated with cortisone derivatives or other immuno-suppressant drugs. Thirdly, when rats are infected in early life, they harbour *Nippostrongylus* for a longer period than when infected as young adults. In this case, we must assume that the neonatal hosts have not developed full immuno-competence and perhaps are not able to recognize and respond to the antigen at the beginning of the infection as effectively as do the older hosts. *Nippostrongylus* has also been found to live for a longer time in lactating rats than in nulliparous females.

We now know that a multi-component immune mechanism brings about the expulsion of *Nippostrongylus*, but not all the steps in the process have been confirmed unequivocally. Humoral antibody is involved in the rat's response, but its activity does not account for all the events that occur. Although some rats with no previous experience of *Nippostrongylus* may be immunized by the passive transfer of serum from an immune donor, the technique is not always successful. Antibody against *Nippostrongylus* can be detected in the serum of neonatal and lactating rats which are known to be harbouring the worms, but the characteristic expulsion of the worms (fig. 9.10) does not occur. These antibodies are undoubtedly protective in function, and ultrastructural studies on adult *Nippostrongylus* have demonstrated changes which can be correlated with the secretion of antibody by the host. For example, the production of gametes becomes abnormal and spermatozoa are re-absorbed in the male reproductive tract, while the cytoplasm of the intestinal epithelial cells becomes electron dense and droplets of lipid accumulate in the hypodermis and muscles of the body wall. All these signs show that disintegration of the tissues is occurring. In the immune rats, third-stage larvae are immobilized within 2 or 3 hours of penetrating the skin, the larval cuticle is seen to be damaged and breakdown of the underlying hypodermis and muscles follows in sequence. Although adult worms are attacked in this way by antibody, the fact that they are not expelled from neonatal and lactating rats indicates that some other factor or factors may contribute to expulsion.

Enough has been said already to show that the thymus gland, which is essential for cell-mediated immunity (fig. 9.1), is concerned with the response of rats to *Nippostrongylus*. Most workers believe that a cellular response contributes to the expulsion of those worms which have been damaged by antibody. Examination of tissue reactions of the rat's intestinal wall indicates that many leukocytes congregate there during the course of the infection. Rats which have been immuno-suppressed by X-rays cannot be protected from *Nippostrongylus* unless they are also given lymph-node cells from normal rats which have not been irradiated. If worms which are known to have been damaged by antibody action are surgically transferred to irradiated rats, they are not expelled after the appropriate time interval (fig. 9.10) unless lymph-node cells from similar non-irradiated rats are transferred also.

With the exception of *Nippostrongylus, Trichinella spiralis* and *Schistosoma mansoni* (see below), there is little detailed information about the immune responses of vertebrate hosts to parasitic worms. The published literature contains many observations which suggest that various species of worm may provoke immune responses. Amongst the nematodes, *Ascaris, Ancylostoma caninum* and *Trichostrongylus colubriformis* stimulate protective immunity. The liver fluke, *Fasciola*, may live for 11 years in experimentally infected sheep, but for not more than a year in cattle. In young calves, primary exposure to 750 metacercariae (fig. 3.36) induced resistance strong enough to destroy about 80% of a challenge infection 17 weeks later. Relatively little is known about how immunity affects tapeworms and even less is known about the responses of vertebrates to acanthocephalans. Those tapeworms which develop in the tissue of vertebrate intermediate hosts usually generate some form of immune response, whereas those tapeworms which live mainly in the lumen of the small intestine may be in a site where immuno-competent cells cannot readily intervene. *Hymenolepis* grows to a considerable size in rats, but survives for a time in mice as a tiny tapeworm. In immuno-suppressed mice, however, *Hymenolepis* grows to maturity. The immediate implications of this observation are that (*a*) the tapeworm and the rat are very closely adapted so that the rat's immune system does not recognize the worm as not-self; (*b*) in the mouse, the tapeworm is recognized and its growth is kept in check by some form of immune response; (*c*) in the immuno-suppressed mouse, the response is either absent or incomplete or ineffective and thus the parasite is able to flourish.

### 9.2.3. *Allergic reactivity to parasitic worms*

The hypersensitive responses of the host's immune system to parasitic worms contribute to the severity of many parasitic diseases and to the form of lesions which are observed. The eggs of *Schistosoma mansoni* (fig. 3.2) and *S. japonicum* gradually accumulate in the liver and other tissues, which react by granuloma formation (fig. 9.11). A granuloma develops as the result of the cellular infiltration of eosinophilic leukocytes and other white cells. Ultimately, fibrous tissue and calcification may replace the cells of the granuloma and the tissue concerned is thus irreparably damaged. Procedures like neonatal thymectomy, which suppresses cell-mediated immunity, almost eliminate granuloma formation. During the course of an experimental infection with *S. mansoni*, the host becomes more sensitized to the eggs and an accelerated granulomatous response

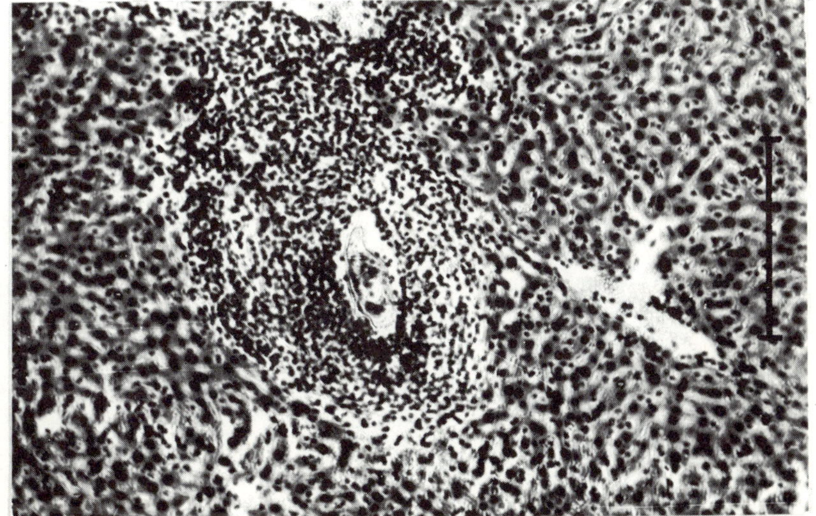

Fig. 9.11. A section through a granuloma formed in the liver of a mouse around an egg of *Schistosoma mansoni* (Digenea). The scale represents approximately 150 $\mu$m.

occurs as more eggs arrive in the liver or other tissue. Thus, we might expect the rate of tissue damage to be accelerated so that the host is more likely to die. Once again, however, the course of evolution seems to have produced some form of equilibrium. In mice which had been treated so that granulomas did not develop, areas of liquefaction and necrosis appeared around the eggs of *Schistosoma* in the liver, and such infected mice did not live as long as those which produced granulomas. The granuloma seems to shield the liver from the effects of toxic factors released by the eggs.

Infections of *Ascaris* in man may be complicated and made more serious by a host response which resembles systemic anaphylaxis, in which certain types of leukocytes known as mast cells (fig. 9.12) are involved. Mast cells become sensitized with antibodies which belong to the class of immunoglobulins known as IgE. On making contact with antigen, the mast cells rupture to release active amines which bring about violent spasms in smooth muscles. Usually, systemic anaphylaxis occurs in appropriately sensitized people after certain insect bites or injections of penicillin and, in highly sensitized or allergic subjects, it is only a timely dose of adrenaline that prevents rapid death from asphyxia. Antibodies of the IgE class are also produced in response to the presence of several endoparasitic worms; as yet no protective function is known for these antibodies. A recent

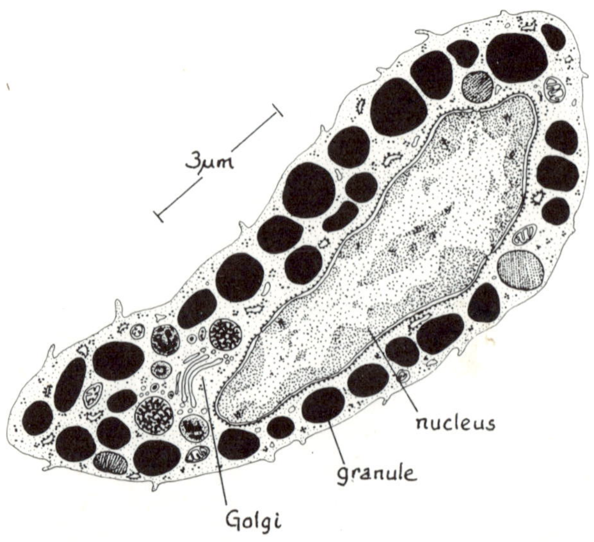


Fig. 9.12. Interpretation, based on electron micrographs, of the structure of a mast cell. These leukocytes manufacture pharmacological active amines which are stored in granules (after Lentz, 1971, *Cell Fine Structure*).

study of young Nigerian children who died suddenly for unknown reasons showed that 96% of them were infected with *Ascaris*. Degranulated mast cells (this is cytological jargon for recording that the mast cells had discharged their amines) were found throughout the cadavers and the conclusion that the children died from unrecognized anaphylaxis seems not at all unreasonable. The development of *Ascaris* gives plenty of opportunity for sensitization to occur as the larval stages wander around the body. During infections with *Trichinella spiralis*, the signs and symptoms of the host–parasite relationship include fever, urticaria (nettle rash) and peri-orbital oedema; all these conditions are usually associated with hypersensitivity.

## 9.3. *Evasion of the immune response*

All kinds of parasites, in addition to worms, may survive for weeks, months or even years in immuno-competent hosts (see table 8.1 for details of worm longevity). How does a natural host–parasite relationship achieve for the parasite the immunological acceptance which eludes all the skills of transplant surgeons? In some cases partial failure or temporary ineffectiveness of the hosts' responses may occur. In other cases, factors intrinsic to the parasite may have evolved which enable it to evade or impede the immunological attack. Defects in the hosts' responses may (*a*) have a genetic basis, (*b*) be related to the age and developmental stage of the host, as in the case of *Nippostrongylus* in neonatal and lactating rats, (*c*) result from the immuno-suppressive effects of other parasitic organisms, (*d*) be related to nutrition, and (*e*) involve enhancing antibodies. Results from research into mammalian embryology have demonstrated that when a mouse of one strain has borne several successive litters to a male of a different strain the survival of skin grafts from the paternal strain is prolonged. It is thought that the graft becomes coated with a layer of harmless antibody which blocks the rejection response. The presence of the blocking antibodies seems to enhance the survival of the graft. Perhaps an analogous condition may sometimes arise in particular host–parasite relationships.

Several lines of evidence have indicated that at least three types of intrinsic mechanism could enable parasites to survive in an immunologically hostile environment. First, a parasite might live in a site where the capacity of the host to respond is reduced or where access for humoral factors is difficult. Secondly, a parasite might stay one step ahead of the host's antibody response by variation of its antigens. Imagine a parasite which released antigen A, followed by B, C and others, at intervals which ensured that by the time antibody A was produced, antigen A had disappeared and had been replaced by B. Antibody B would now be synthesized, but would not be able to combine with antigen C and so on. Thirdly, a parasite may present a surface which the host cannot identify as not-self; the parasite is masquerading in some way as host tissue.

Most is known about how *Schistosoma mansoni* might survive in a host which is responding to its presence. A rather simplified representation of what appears to happen in rhesus monkeys is shown in fig. 9.13. When a rhesus monkey is infected for the first time with cercariae of *Schistosoma*, a patent infection develops. Subsequent attempts to infect the monkey fail and new blood flukes are not added to the resident population. Similar observations can be made with *Schistosoma* in mice. Antibodies and host cells kill the invading stages of the secondary infection, but not the established worms. Adult worms have been taken from monkeys and implanted surgically into the mesenteric veins of similar recipient monkeys which have not had any previous experience of *Schistosoma*. The recipient monkeys also develop powerful immunity against subsequent infections, but not against the worms which were transplanted. This form of immunity is now called concomitant immunity. One obvious biological effect is that the first worms to become established in an environment where space may be a limiting resource may have little trouble from competitors.

Clues about the immunological mechanisms of concomitant immunity were obtained when adults of *Schistosoma* were transplanted directly from mice to rhesus monkeys. The worms took some time to adjust to the new host and there was a delay before egg production restarted. Nevertheless, those worms which became established elicited responses typical of concomitant immunity. If worms from mice were transplanted into monkeys which had been immunized against the tissues of the donor mice, the worms were rapidly destroyed. These results indicated that the adult worms, of either a natural or an artificial primary infection, had in some manner acquired a surface which the immune responses of the host did not detect or could not attack. The transplantation of worms from mice into normal and immunized monkeys suggested that in the former case the mouse worms took time to change their surfaces from mouse to monkey and that in the latter case there was insufficient time to make the change. The death of the mouse worms in the immunized monkeys supports the view that the mouse worms were disguised as mouse.

*Schistosoma mansoni* can now be maintained *in vitro*, and growth occurs provided that the appropriate type of serum is present in the incubation medium. The method of promoting the growth of *Schistosoma in vitro* consists of allowing cercariae to penetrate a skin membrane and enter a chamber containing the nutrient medium. In this way, the cercarial tail is lost and the transformation to the schistosomulum is achieved. An important result from this technique is that the young schistosomulum is killed *in vitro* if the serum has been prepared from a host harbouring living adult *Schistosoma*. Similarly, worms grown *in vitro* with human serum are killed on surgical transplantation into monkeys, if the monkeys have been immunized against the same serum or against the erythrocytes of the

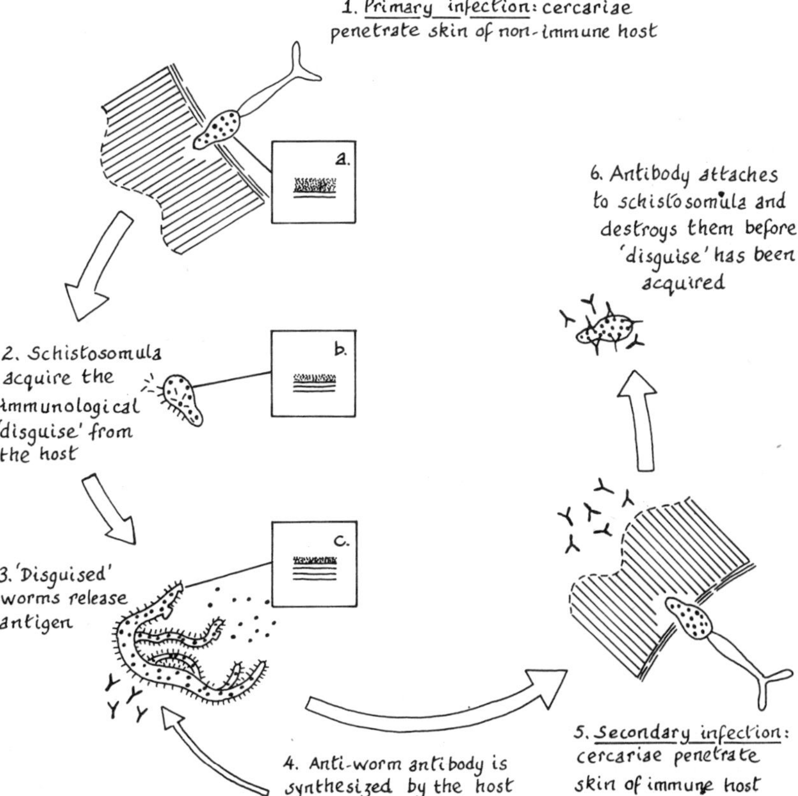


Fig. 9.13. Diagrammatic presentation of a hypothesis concerning some of the immunological relationships of *Schistosoma mansoni* (Digenea) with a definitive host. The inserts (a–c) show surface membranes of the parasite (after Terry and Smithers, 1975).

donor who provided the serum. An extension of this approach has shown that antigens of the A, B and O blood groups can be incorporated into the surface of the young schistosomulum and that these might well provide the necessary disguise. The theory becomes even more attractive because complex and rapid changes occur at the surface of *Schistosoma* developing in the definitive host (fig. 9.13). The changes in the surface membranes might present a suitable substrate for the incorporation of host antigens. In the case of concomitant immunity, it is assumed that antibody is able to damage the schistosomula before the disguise of host antigen has been adopted.

We must stop at this point: all research scientists soon realize that caution is necessary when hypotheses and theories are derived to fit observations and even more caution is needed if results obtained under one set of conditions are to be extrapolated and applied to fit another set. For example, can we be confident that what happens at the surface of *Schistosoma in vitro* also happens *in vivo*? How can we know that we have not ignored other mechanisms and factors which contribute to the evasion of the host response by *Schistosoma*? We have seen that vertebrate hosts have the capacity to synthesize a vast range of antibody molecules. Perhaps *Schistosoma*, and other species of endoparasitic worm, can synthesize molecules to deceive their hosts or inactivate their hosts' mechanisms of resistance. This whole area of research may prove to be most rewarding; if more progress is made, vaccines may be produced to relieve human suffering and misery.

# 10. Worms and man

The writings of our ancestors reveal that from ancient times man has suffered from parasitic worms. *Ascaris* was obviously a problem for earlier civilizations from China to Peru. Not surprisingly, our ancestors were bedevilled by ignorance and some of their ideas about diagnosis and treatment appear absurd. A physician would wrap a fish in a bandage around a patient's abdomen; and if the fish was eaten, he would conclude that his patient had worms. Chinese prescriptions for the removal of worms often involved the ash of human hair, bits of dried toad, the blood of pigs, chicken manure and the salts of heavy metals. Some of these preparations were no doubt very efficacious, although the unfortunate patient may have suffered from undesirable side-effects. Ignorance, not only of facts but also of scientific and medical methods, is still a major obstacle in attempts to relieve and control helminth disease.

A disease is a derangement of health or a disordered condition of a tissue or organism. Infectious diseases, including those associated with parasitic worms, involve the transmission of an agent from one animal to another. The development of a disease, however, depends on many factors in addition to those which influence the establishment and growth of infectious agents in suitable hosts. Apart from a community's unavoidable ecological overlap with a given parasite, the social customs, agricultural practices, education, economic position and nutritional status of the people influence the development of a disease. Nutrition seems to be a very important factor. Many parasitic diseases flourish in the areas of the world where people suffer from hunger and undernutrition. Nutritional deficiencies appear to reduce antibody synthesis, phagocytic activity, inflammatory responses and the effectiveness of natural barriers to infection. In addition, the presence of an endoparasite may interfere with the food intake and digestion of the host and so contribute to the state of undernutrition. Once people experience chronic undernutrition, they are not usually able to increase their productivity to acquire sufficient funds to improve sanitation, build hospitals or buy insecticides and drugs. Furthermore, the lack of a potential market may prevent pharmaceutical companies in more prosperous countries from investing capital in the development of drugs. All these factors, some of which are considered briefly below, are connected and interdependent; parasitic disease should always be considered as a highly complex subject.

## 10.1. *Prevalence of helminth infections in man*

At least 70 species of parasitic worm are known to infect man. Several of these are rare or accidental and of little consequence to a population as a whole. Recent estimations of the prevalence of worms of medical importance are given in table 10.1. Most of these affect people living in the developing countries of tropical and subtropical

TABLE 10.1. *Endoparasitic worms of medical importance with estimates of their prevalence (after Peters and Gilles, 1977).*

| Species | Prevalence (millions of cases) |
|---|---|
| DIGENEA | |
| *Clonorchis sinensis* | 28 |
| *Paragonimus westermani* | 5 |
| *Schistosoma haematobium* 78 | |
| *S. japonicum* 69 | 204 |
| *S. mansoni* 57 | |
| CESTODA | |
| *Diphyllobothrium latum* | 13 |
| *Hymenolepis nana* | 29 |
| *Taenia saginata* | 61 |
| *T. solium* | 4 |
| NEMATODA | |
| *Ascaris lumbricoides* | 986 |
| *Dracunculus medinensis* | 79 |
| *Enterobius vermicularis* | 291 |
| Hookworm (*Ancylostoma duodenale* and *Necator americanus*) | 716 |
| *Loa loa* | 26 |
| *Onchocerca volvulus* | 39 |
| *Trichinella spiralis* | 39 |
| *Trichuris trichiura* | 536 |
| *Wuchereria bancrofti* and *Brugia malayi* | 296 |
| Total | 3352 |

regions. Since the world's population is about 4000 million and many people in temperate climates are free of worms, the information in table 10.1 implies that some people may harbour more than one species of worm. Multiple infections are common, *Ascaris, Trichuris, Schistosoma* and hookworms being frequently found together. Many of the millions of hosts listed in the table are unlikely to show the signs and symptoms of illness. Their infections will be light and they will not be diseased, although they will serve to disseminate infective stages into the environment and so ensure the survival of parasites which in other people may become established in dangerously high numbers. Even where most infections are light, health workers with experience of life in a tropical village consider that the well-being of many people would be improved if endoparasitic worms could be eliminated. Parasitic worms also thrive in and damage domestic animals and thus deprive man of food and even of his livelihood.

The suffix '-iasis'† is generally combined with the name of a worm to indicate a host–parasite relationship in which disease may develop. For example, infections with *Ascaris* and *Schistosoma* are referred to as ascariasis and schistosomiasis respectively. Some authors use the suffix '-iosis' to denote a condition of disease. In this book '-iasis' has normally been used regardless of the state of balance between a host and its parasite.

## 10.2. *Human behaviour and helminth disease*

### 10.2.1. *Transmission and infection*

During the evolution of his cultural and social life, man has unwittingly adopted many practices which have favoured the spread of parasites. For example, schistosomiasis depends on contact between man and water containing susceptible snails. Water contamination and exposure to infection are inherent in irrigation and agriculture, and in domestic, recreational and religious behaviour. In a study of the pattern of water-contact activities of villagers in a region of Egypt where schistosomiasis is a major health hazard, the people were observed to experience thirteen types of water-contact activity (table 10.2). The workers concluded that females had more frequent contacts with water than did males, and that males were responsible for more contamination than the females. Most water contact occurred in summer, and the washing of dishes and kitchen utensils was one of the commonest activities during the time of day when

† The first *i* is long (as in eye) and accented.

TABLE 10.2. *Observations on the frequency of outdoor social and religious water-contact activities in an Egyptian rural area (after Farooq and Mallah, 1966,* Bull. Wld. Hlth. Org. **35,** *377).*

| Contact activity | Number of activities in age-groups (years): Boys and men | | | | | Girls and women | | | | |
|---|---|---|---|---|---|---|---|---|---|---|
| | 0–9 | 10–14 | 15–24 | 25+ | total | 0–9 | 10–14 | 15–24 | 25+ | total |
| Washing clothes | — | — | — | 3 | 3 | 3 | 31 | 57 | 63 | 154 |
| Washing utensils | — | 2 | — | — | 2 | 267 | 173 | 192 | 236 | 868 |
| Washing animals | 3 | 11 | 33 | 18 | 65 | 1 | 3 | 6 | 10 | 20 |
| Washing vegetables | — | 2 | 5 | 4 | 11 | 1 | 1 | — | — | 2 |
| Bathing and playing | 323 | 20 | 7 | 6 | 356 | 247 | — | 3 | 7 | 257 |
| Swimming | 12 | 9 | — | — | 21 | — | — | — | — | — |
| Urination | 8 | — | 10 | 16 | 34 | 4 | — | — | 1 | 5 |
| Defaecation and urination | 17 | — | 4 | 26 | 47 | 11 | — | — | — | 11 |
| Ablution[a] | 3 | 1 | 8 | 40 | 52 | 2 | — | — | — | 2 |
| Wadu[b] | — | 2 | 15 | 71 | 88 | — | — | — | — | — |
| Taking water | 1 | 1 | — | 4 | 6 | 14 | 30 | 70 | 105 | 219 |
| Angling | 13 | 9 | — | 1 | 23 | — | — | — | — | — |
| Net fishing | — | — | — | 2 | 2 | — | — | — | — | — |

[a] Ablution is the washing of the anal and peri-anal region after defaecation. Ablution is performed mainly by males who squat close to the water's edge and wash with the left hand.

[b] Wadu is the ritual washing enjoined by religion on adult male Muslims before prayers, which are said five times a day.

most infective cercariae were at large. Schistosomiasis might become a minor problem if each home in an endemic region could be provided with a sink, a clean water supply and a lavatory.

Among the filarial nematodes, *Onchocerca volvulus* (table 10.1) has devastated the health of many people in tropical West Africa. The worm is transmitted by black fly (*Simulium damnosum* complex) which develop in streams and rivers. Onchocerciasis produces severe, chronic itching, disfiguring changes in the skin, and damage to the eye which may culminate in blindness. Man may have contributed to his present plight by penetrating into the semi-arid savannas of West Africa and clearing the vegetation around the water-ways in order to grow and irrigate his crops. *Simulium damnosum* is an insect catholic in its choice of hosts for blood meals, but dependent on living near water for breeding. Clearance of the bush and the establishment of agriculture probably drove away nearly all the food for *Simulium* and left man, with an equal need to live near the water, as the main source of blood. Other misfortunes have befallen man. The biting flies *Chrysops silacea* and *C. dimidiata*, which transmit *Loa loa* (table 10.1) in West Africa, have been found to be attracted to wood smoke.

Some of our habits and customs may have helped to protect us from parasitic disease. In the Mosaic law, the classification of animals into clean and unclean and the prohibition of contact with scavenger animals must have protected communities from many types of parasitic infection.

### 10.2.2. *Man and animals*

There are numerous records of man naturally acquiring parasitic worms which normally live and grow in other vertebrate hosts. Infections of this type are known as zoonoses and some are very important. *Trichinella spiralis* attains maturity in the small intestine of rats and small carnivorous mammals. The adult female worm releases first-stage larvae which pass through the intestinal wall and eventually become encysted in a characteristic form in the host's muscles (fig. 3.43), the life cycle being maintained by cannibalistic, predatory and scavenging habits. Thus, larger animals like bears and pigs may become infected, and man becomes vulnerable if he eats under-cooked pork from pig farms where unsatisfactory standards of hygiene exist (table 10.1). The migrations of the larvae of *T. spiralis* are often accompanied by marked irritation, oedema, fever, pain and cardiac and pulmonary disturbances. Muscles containing many encysted larvae do not function as well as uninfected tissues.

The relationship between man and domestic dogs has generated much work for the parasitologist (4.3.1). In Kenya, the Masai and the Turkana are two nomadic tribes which depend on cattle and keep dogs to help control their flocks and herds. The dogs are hosts of the tapeworm *Echinococcus granulosus*, which develops as a hydatid cyst in ruminants and sometimes in man (figs. 2.3, 3.35). Hydatid disease is rare among the Masai and common among the Turkana, presumably because the Masai keep their dogs at a distance whereas the Turkana encourage intimate contact with theirs. Turkana dogs may act as nurses for young children and even lick up the mess when the baby vomits and defecates. Thus close relationships are formed between children and dogs, with the result that the eggs of *Echinococcus* are easily transmitted and hydatid cysts develop.

Man's need to keep animals for food has also presented the parasitologist with many problems. The eggs of *Dictyocaulus viviparus* are released by the adult worms in the lungs of cattle and, by the time they have passed up the trachea and over into the oesophagus, many have hatched, releasing first-stage larvae. The larvae pass out of the host in the faeces and develop on the pasture to form infective, ensheathed third-stage larvae, which cattle acquire when contaminated grass is swallowed. Exsheathment occurs in the alimentary tract and the larvae bore through the intestinal wall and reach the lungs where their development is completed. In calves, heavy primary infections of *D. viviparus* often give rise to pneumonia and bronchitis because many of the eggs become trapped in the alveoli of the lungs. Sick cattle are unprofitable and bring the farmer no return on his outlay. The cattle rarely die and, when they recover they can be shown to have developed an effective form of immunity. Under natural conditions or primitive methods of animal husbandry, cattle would not be overcrowded and dependent on nutritional supplements as they are today. They would remain with their mothers for longer than at present and weaning and the change to a grass diet would occur gradually. The fact that the cattle would not have been kept at a high density would mean that the pasture would not carry high numbers of infective larvae. Furthermore, the calves would take small amounts of grass during natural weaning and would thus acquire small numbers of larvae which would elicit immunity with the minimum of disease. Unfortunately, those employed in trying to meet our demands for milk and beef cannot afford the time to allow immunity to develop naturally.

### 10.3. *Pathology*

Some of the signs, symptoms and disorders of certain diseases involving helminths are described below. Only hosts with heavy infections will suffer severe illness or death as the result of parasitic disease. For many people, however, the combined effect of three or more infections results in a lowered standard of health, and a denial of their right to develop fully their physical and mental faculties. A detailed view of the extent of helminth disease can be found in any of the many texts on tropical and veterinary medicine.

#### 10.3.1. *Ascariasis*

The first phase of the disease is associated with the tissue migrations of the larval stages, which are probably most dangerous if many reach the lungs simultaneously. The host develops an asthmatic cough, and suffers from haemorrhage and a form of pneumonia, which may be accompanied by fever and pain. Recently, physicians in North America had an unsolicited opportunity to study this aspect of ascariasis when four university students became seriously ill after eating a festive meal which had been maliciously seasoned with large numbers of infective eggs of *Ascaris*. The body tends to combat the larval *Ascaris* by means of eösinophilic leukocytes, which infiltrate the lungs and other invaded organs. Many of the parasites become immobilized and encapsulated by the host cells; the resulting tiny patches of scar tissue may be very detrimental if the larvae have been caught in the central nervous system.

The second phase of the disease concerns the adult worms in the lumen of the alimentary tract. In young children, the abdomen may be greatly distended when many worms are present, and nausea, vomiting, pain and sleeplessness are common symptoms. The worms also interfere with alimentary functioning. The lumen of the small intestine may be blocked or restricted so that the flow of chyme is impeded. Sometimes a worm may become lodged in the common bile duct or trapped in the appendix. *Ascaris* has been found to secrete substances which inhibit trypsin and chymotrypsin. When jejunal biopsies have been carried out on infected children in hospitals, their intestinal villi, from the region where the *Ascaris* were living, have been found to be inflamed, and to be broader and shorter than those from uninfected children. Alteration of the mucosal structure in this way usually leads to an impairment of the absorption of digestion products. Several studies have shown that children infected with *Ascaris* lose much more nitrogen per day in their faeces than they do after successful treatment of the infection. The effects of *Ascaris* are probably most serious in the many infants whose diet is barely sufficient to support a normal rate of growth. In very heavy infections, growth may be dramatically retarded or the worms may burst through the intestinal wall and enter the abdominal cavity, causing peritonitis. There is a record of about 2000 *Ascaris* having been removed from the body cavity of a young Chinese woman. An effect of an experimental infection of *Ascaris* on the growth of a pig is shown in fig. 10.1.

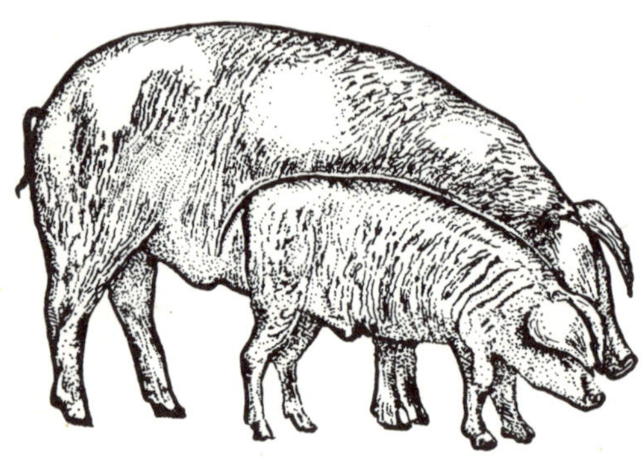

Fig. 10.1. A drawing, based on a photograph, of two litter-mate pigs. The larger pig was reared free from *Ascaris* (Nematoda) and the smaller was heavily infected (after Jones, 1967, *Introduction to Parasitology*).

### 10.3.2. *Hookworm disease*

The hookworms, *Ancylostoma duodenale* and *Necator americanus*, are known to suck blood from the intestinal mucosa, and further blood loss occurs from the damaged tissue which has been chewed and then abandoned by the worms. Hookworms are widespread (table 10.1) and the conclusion is inescapable that many people who suffer from iron-deficient anaemia do so because they are infected with either *Ancylostoma* or *Necator* or both species of nematode.

Iron-deficient anaemia leads to a decrease in the haemoglobin content of the blood and so has numerous indirect effects on health. Men are often considered anaemic if their haemoglobin level falls below 14 g per 100 ml of blood and their erythrocyte count is less than 4.5 million cells per cubic millimetre. In women, these values are usually taken to be 12 g and 4 million cells respectively. The age and physiological condition of a person, the altitude at which he or she lives and the methods used to make the measurements must not be overlooked in any definition of iron-deficient anaemia.

The relationship between the number of hookworms in a host and the development of anaemia is very complex, as has been implied in Chapter 5. The activities of the worms may give rise to a syndrome of malabsorption of iron; the absorption of iron is a relatively inefficient process which is bound to be affected by the dietary iron intake and the endogenous iron reserves of the host. In tropical countries, where hookworm disease is common, iron absorption from the small intestine may be further hampered by the fibre content and phytate concentration of the largely vegetable diet of many people. Some of the iron which is lost during haemorrhage in one part of the small intestine may be reabsorbed in another part, and this recycling of the iron which is already in the body complicates attempts to measure the relationship between hookworm infection and iron-deficient anaemia. Nevertheless, some useful studies have been made and it has been found that in Venezuela people from rural communities are likely to suffer from anaemia if their faeces contain more than 2000 eggs per gram (fig. 10.2).

The symptoms of iron-deficient anaemia include weakness, susceptibility to fatigue, irritability, euphoria, drowsiness, psychotic behaviour, vertigo and headache. Communities cannot be expected to be productive if individuals are in such a state. Any infection causing blood loss will have a tendency to cause anaemia, which often develops in domestic animals infected with large numbers of trichostrongyle nematodes, for example *Haemonchus contortus*. When haemorrhage occurs, however, blood plasma and proteins are lost in addition to red cells, haemoglobin and iron. This condition of hypoalbuminaemia can be as debilitating as iron-deficient anaemia, especially if the host is undernourished and short of protein.

A discussion of worms and anaemia would not be complete without reference to the broad tapeworm, *Diphyllobothrium latum* (fig. 2.3). In the Baltic countries, man acquires the worm from partially-cooked freshwater fish. In some hosts, the production of red cells becomes so abnormal that people appear to be suffering from pernicious anaemia, the disease which develops in people who no longer possess the means of absorbing vitamin $B_{12}$ from the intestine into the bloodstream. Remission of the disease caused by *D. latum* is brought about by the removal of the worm, since it absorbs nearly all the vitamin $B_{12}$ that is ingested by the host.

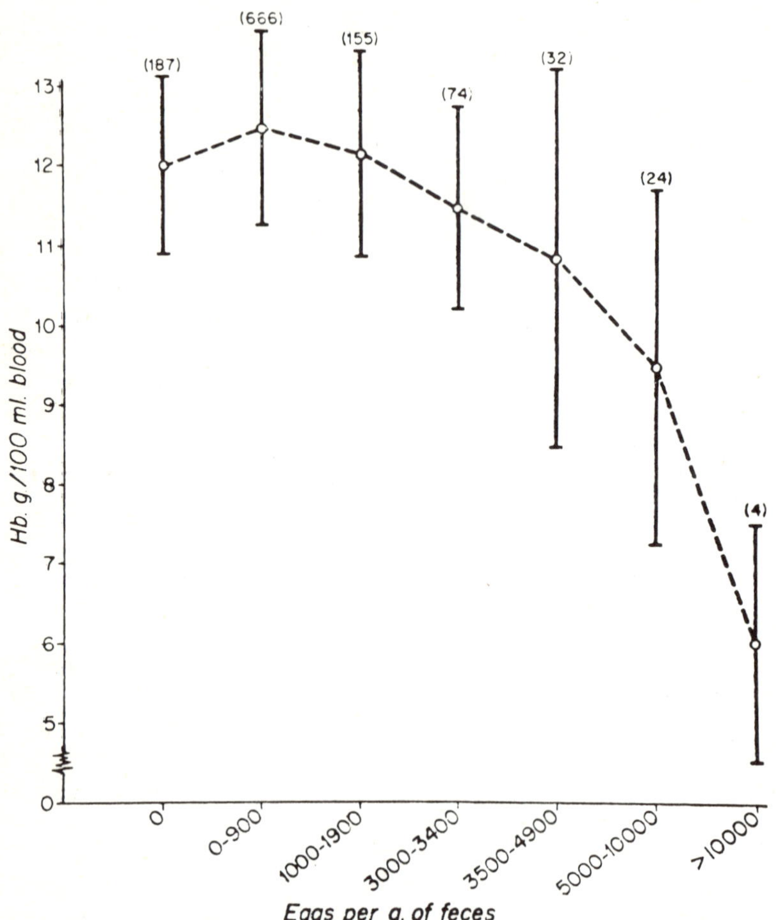


Fig. 10.2. The relationship between haemoglobin levels and the severity of hookworm (Nematoda) infection in various Venezuelan rural communities. The number of cases in each group is shown in parentheses. Vertical lines indicate the standard deviation. In all groups with more than 2000 eggs per gram of faeces, the difference from the negative group is statistically significant ($P<0.01$) (from Roche and Layrisse, 1966, *Am. J. trop. med. Hyg.*, **15**, 1029).

### 10.3.3. *Filariasis*

The effects of filarial nematodes on man are varied. Mention of *Onchocerca volvulus* (table 10.1) has already been made (10.2.1). Its microfilarial stages, which are responsible for most features of the disease, live mainly in the skin and their arrival in the eye leads to the loss of vision known as river blindness. In some parts of Africa, over 10% of the population are blind and another 20% have impaired eyesight. There are reckoned to be about 70 000 adults with 'economic blindness' in the upper Volta basin.

The adult stages of *Wuchereria bancrofti* (table 10.1) initiate the condition known as elephantiasis† (fig. 10.3). Masses of worms obstruct the lymphatics, so that in a matter of years hideous swellings arise from the accumulation of excess fluids and host tissue. Conditions as advanced as that illustrated in fig. 10.3 are rarely seen nowadays, although some degree of swelling is common. The disease has long been present in India. In the Indian Medical Gazette of 1902, an army surgeon described his technique for removing the 'tumours'. One growth was reckoned to weigh 'quite 100 lbs . . . It enclosed a double hydrocoele, each containing a large quantity of fluid, and the serous drain from the elephantoid tissue during the operation was very copious. The contents of the tunical sacs rose in a fountain over our heads directly the knife punctured them'.

### 10.3.4. *Schistosomiasis*

Schistosomiasis is a chronic condition which develops when the spiny eggs of the flukes become trapped in the host's tissues during heavy infections (9.2.3). When eggs of *Schistosoma mansoni* and *S. japonicum* are released by the female worms, some pass through the intestinal wall and are carried out of the host, some are trapped in the tissues of the intestine and some are carried into the liver and other organs by the flow of blood in the veins of the portal system. The tissues of the lower intestine are damaged both by the encapsulation and calcification of trapped eggs and by the passage of free ones. Intestinal haemorrhage may occur and contribute to a state of anaemia in the host. The greater the number of eggs in the liver, the less is the hepatic tissue available for normal metabolic functions. Eventually, so much of the liver may have been irritated that the walls of the hepatic blood vessels become calcified, and the condition known as clay pipe-stem fibrosis sets in. The presence of the infection also interferes with the flow of blood in the hepatic portal system.

† The name 'elephantiasis' refers to the appearance of the disease, not to infection with elephants.

The human host may harbour *S. mansoni* for a long time without showing any obvious signs and symptoms of disease. The information given in table 10.3 was obtained from 69 people who were classified as asymptomatic until the post-mortem examination was carried out. *Schistosoma mansoni* is usually considered to be a less serious pathogen than *S. japonicum*, the females of which appear to produce about ten times as many eggs per day as an equivalent number of females of *S. mansoni*. One commentator has claimed that a massive and rapid outbreak of schistosomiasis (*S. japonicum*) in Mao Tse-Tung's army in 1949 saved Formosa from invasion. When man is infected with *S. haematobium*, the disease is caused by eggs becoming trapped in the walls of the ureters and bladder. A great deal of tissue damage and haemorrhage occurs, cystitis is common and the patient has problems with urination. In women, some eggs may become lodged in the ovaries, fallopian tubes and uterine wall.

## 10.4. *Economic aspects of helminth disease*

Parasitologists have concluded that control programmes against relatively unspectacular chronic diseases need to be presented as

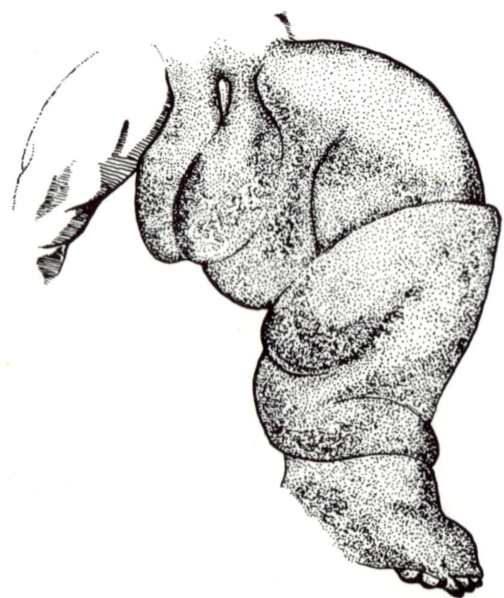

Fig. 10.3. A drawing of an extreme case of elephantiasis in which excess tissue has developed after blockage of the lymph vessels by adult *Wuchereria bancrofti* (Nematoda) (after Jones, 1967).

TABLE 10.3. *Observations made at post mortem examination on infections of* Schistosoma mansoni *(Digenea) in Brazil (after Cheever, 1968).*

| | | Mean number of eggs | | | |
|---|---|---|---|---|---|
| Number of cadavers examined | Number of worm pairs per cadaver[a] | Per liver | Per liver per worm pair | Per g faeces | Per g faeces per worm pair |
| 18 | 1–5 | 26 900 | 14 900 | 56 | 22 |
| 19 | 6–10 | 44 400 | 6 100 | 91 | 11 |
| 11 | 11–20 | 97 500 | 5 100 | 296 | 20 |
| 11 | 21–40 | 100 400 | 3 700 | 452 | 22 |
| 10 | 41–80 | 225 600 | 4 000 | 317 | 6 |

[a] Worm pairs were obtained from the cadavers by perfusion of the hepatic portal system.

profitable enterprises in order to attract financial support and to give them their due place in the list of priorities which governments must consider in the use of their available funds. Several attempts have been made to estimate the economic losses associated with schistosomiasis. In the early 1950s, the productivity of Egypt was thought to be reduced by about a third and 24 million man hours were lost in Japan as a result of schistosome infections. In 1972, the various forms of the disease were endemic in 71 countries and about 1400 million people were at risk. A very conservative estimate suggested that schistosomiasis resulted in a resource loss of about $642 million (about £260 million); this figure did not include the costs of sickness benefits, pensions, treatment schemes and so on. Some agencies and governments are now investigating worker productivity and parasitic infections in detail. A team tries to determine the cost-to-benefit ratio from providing a drug or nutritional supplement for a sample of a labour force, while measuring the increase in net profit which is generated by the efforts of those affected by the intervention. If a low expenditure on drugs or nutrients is found to lead to a marked increase in productivity, many industrialists and governments will have difficult decisions to make and new problems to face.

## 10.5. *Control*

Attempts to control parasitic infections may be by physical, chemical and biological methods. Physical methods include schemes designed to introduce or improve domestic and community water supplies and sewage disposal. The building of bridges and roads and the provision of protective clothing serve to reduce the exposure of people to water-borne infections. Chemical methods involve the use of disinfectants, molluscicides, insecticides and drugs. Any chemical should be used with great caution and only after much research, as environmental contamination may lead to disastrous consequences for the local flora and fauna. Resistant strains of intermediate host and vector may emerge in response to the use of chemicals. According to the World Health Organization, 35 species of insect were known to be resistant to insecticide in 1958 and 74 more species were resistant by 1971. Drugs must also be used with care and under proper supervision. The perfect drug for use against helminth disease in tropical populations, when funds, medical workers and other facilities are in short supply, is very rare (6.5).

Biological methods of control depend on the action of parasites, predators and pathogens in lowering another organism's population density. In theory, the vectors, intermediate hosts and free-living stages of helminths should be vulnerable to this form of attack, but the introduction of a control organism should not be contemplated until sufficient knowledge is available about the population dynamics of the prime target and the potential targets in the region. The use of vaccines can also be considered as one of the methods of biological control. At present, attenuated third-stage larvae of *Dictyocaulus viviparus* are given in two doses to cattle in the United Kingdom and very significant protection from disease is obtained. In the laboratory, dogs can be protected from the effects of *Ancylostoma caninum* by a similar procedure. Protection from hookworm disease in man may eventually become available, although the production of a vaccine and its distribution to the millions of people at risk will present a colossal administrative problem.

All the methods for the control of parasitic disease depend on knowledge and education. Research workers must improve our knowledge of parasite biology, host responses and host–parasite interactions. Epidemiologists must study the transmission of disease and develop methods of forecasting when and where outbreaks are likely to occur. Chemists, pharmacologists and clinicians must provide safe and cheap drugs. Governments must consider the position of man's health in their orders of priority for funds. Every individual on the planet is involved, in some way, in this situation and enterprise. Everyone is at risk. Education is the means whereby parasitic disease will be controlled without the destruction of our environment.

# Glossary

Explanations are provided below for some of the terms used in this and other books on parasitology.

*Aetiology*. The study of the agents and factors involved in the causation of disease.

*Anaerobiosis*. Life in the absence or near absence of free oxygen.

*Anatomy*. The science of the arrangement of the parts of the body of an organism.

*Antibody*. A molecule produced by an animal in response to exposure to antigen. Antibody molecules (immunoglobulins) consist mainly of protein and have the property of combining specifically with the antigen.

*Antigen*. A molecule which, under the appropriate conditions, elicits the production of antibody.

*Antiserum*. Serum prepared from an immune animal and known to contain particular antibodies.

*Atrophy*. Diminution in size, or in function, through lack of food or use.

*Autoradiography*. A method of demonstrating the distribution of chemical substances in the tissues by first making them radioactive, then recording their presence on photographic film which has been placed in contact with the treated tissue.

*Cadaver*. A dead human body retained for anatomical or medical investigation.

*Chemotherapy*. The treatment of disease by chemical agents.

*Chyme*. The partially digested food which is passed from the stomach into the small intestine.

*Classification*. The process of defining and arranging organisms into groups. An ideal classification should be a natural one based as far as possible on established evolutionary relationships.

*Clone*. A population of cells (or organisms) of identical genetical constitution derived asexually from a single cell by repeated division.

*Cybernetics*. The science of communication and control.

*Cytochemistry*. The identification and localization of chemical compounds within cells.

*Differentiation*. The process by which cells, tissues or organs gradually change their form and function.

*Dioecious*. Having the sexes separate.

*Disease*. A definite morbid process having characteristic signs and symptoms.

*Epidemiology*. The study of the relationships of the various factors determining the frequency and distribution of diseases in communities.

*Fecundity*. Capacity of an organism (or species) to reproduce.

*Filariform*. Thread-like.

*Hermaphrodite*. An individual possessing functional male and female reproductive organs.

*Histochemistry*. The identification and localization of chemical compounds within tissues.

*Histology*. The study of the microscopic structure of tissues.

*Homoiothermal*. Having a more or less constant body temperature (warm-blooded).

*Hypersensitivity*. A state of increased or exaggerated reactivity to antigen brought about by previous exposure.

*Hypertrophy*. The growth of an organ or organism by increase in cell size rather than cell number.

*Immuno-competence*. The full ability of an organism to respond to contact with antigen. The responsiveness includes the formation of specific antibody and cell-mediated reactions.

*Incidence*. The number of new cases of an infection reported in an area in a unit of time.

*Lesion*. A pathological disturbance of a cell, tissue or organ.

*Metamorphosis*. The change of form and structure undergone by an animal during development.

*Morphology*. The study of the form and structure of an organ or organism.

*Necrosis*. The death of cells, tissues or organs.

*Neonatal*. New-born.

*Neoteny*. The retention of larval characters beyond the normal period. In extreme cases, the animal is able to breed while maintaining its larval or juvenile form.

*Nulliparous*. Never having given birth to a live infant (mammal).

*Parasitaemia*. An estimate of the number of parasites (usually microfilariae in the case of helminthology) in the blood or appropriate tissue of the living host.

*Parthenogenesis*. Reproduction in which the egg or oocyte is activated by a factor(s) other than a spermatozoon.

*Patent period*. The time for which eggs or larval stages are observed to be produced by parasitic worms.

*Pathogenicity*. The capacity of an organism to produce disease.

*Pathology*. The study of the structural and functional changes in cells, tissues and organs which are associated with disease.

*Phylogeny*. The evolutionary relationships and history of groups of organisms.

*Phylum*. A major taxonomic group in which the members share basically similar anatomical features.

*Physiology*. The study of the functions of tissues, organs and organisms in terms of physical and chemical processes.

*Poikilothermal*. Having a body temperature which varies with that of the surrounding medium.

*Polyembryony*. The formation of many individuals, having identical genetic material, from one egg.

*Prepatent period*. The period for which parasitic worms are present in their hosts before the release of eggs or larval stages is first detected.

*Prevalence*. The number of cases of an infection or a disease in existence at a certain time in a designated area.

*Protandry*. A condition of hermaphrodites in which male gametes develop before female gametes.

*Race*. A group of organisms within a species whose members can be distinguished from other members of the species by biochemical, morphological, pathogenic or physiological characteristics but remain capable of breeding with them (synonymous with strain).

*Species*. A group of similar organisms breeding among themselves and not normally with organisms of another group.

*Strain*. Synonymous with race.

*Syncytium*. A multi-nucleate mass of cytoplasm.

*Taxonomy*. The science of the principles and practice of classification.

*Vaccine*. A suspension of dead or living organisms, or their products, which is injected into another organism with the intention of producing a state of immunity.

*Vector*. An intermediate host which serves to carry a parasite to the definitive host.

*Virulence*. A variable pathogenic character(s) of a parasite often determined in part by conditions prevailing in the host.

*Viviparity*. The form of reproduction which is characterized by the mother giving birth to developed young ones.

*Zoonosis*. An infection naturally transmitted between man and other vertebrates.

*Some singular and plural forms:*

| | | | |
|---|---|---|---|
| Acanthella | -llae | Proboscis | -scides |
| Cercaria | -ariae | Proglottis | -ttides |
| Microfilaria | -ariae | Redia | -diae |
| Miracidium | -dia | Schistosomulum | -ula |
| Microthrix | -triches | Scolex | -eces |

'It is not my intention to stick stubbornly to my opinions, but as soon as people urge against them any reasonable objections . . . I'll give mine up and go over to the other side.' Anthony van Leeuwenhoek, 1694.

# Further reading and references

*General Parasitology*

BAER, J. G. (1971). *Animal Parasites*. London: Weidenfeld and Nicolson.

KENNEDY, C. R. (1975). *Ecological Animal Parasitology*. Oxford, London, Edinburgh and Melbourne: Blackwell Scientific Publications.

NNOCHIRI, E. (1975). *Medical Parasitology in the Tropics*. Oxford University Press.

READ, C. P. (1970). *Parasitism and Symbiology*. New York: The Ronald Press.

SCHMIDT, G. D. and ROBERTS, L. S. (1977). *Foundations of Parasitology*. St. Louis: The C. V. Mosby Company.

SMYTH, J. D. (1976). *Introduction to Animal Parasitology*, 2nd edition. London, Sydney, Auckland and Toronto: Hodder and Stoughton.

*Helminthology*

BURT, D. R. R. (1970). *Platyhelminthes and Parasitism*. London: The English Universities Press Limited.

CROLL, N. A. and MATTHEWS, B. E. (1977). *Biology of Nematodes*. Glasgow and London: Blackie.

CROMPTON, D. W. T. (1970). *An Ecological Approach to Acanthocephalan Physiology*. Cambridge University Press.

DAWES, B. (1946). *The Trematoda*. Cambridge University Press.

ERASMUS, D. A. (1972). *The Biology of Trematodes*. London: Edward Arnold.

LEE, D. L. (1965). *The Physiology of Nematodes*. Edinburgh and London: Oliver and Boyd.

LEE, D. L. and ATKINSON, H. J. (1976). *Physiology of Nematodes*, 2nd edition. London and Basingstoke: The Macmillan Press Limited.

LYONS, K. M. (1978). *The Biology of Helminth Parasites*. Studies in Biology No. 102. London: Edward Arnold.

MULLER, R. (1975). *Worms and Disease*. London: William Heinemann Medical Books Limited.

SMYTH, J. D. (1966). *The Physiology of Trematodes*. Edinburgh and London: Oliver and Boyd.

SMYTH, J. D. (1969). *The Physiology of Cestodes*. Edinburgh and London: Oliver and Boyd.

WRIGHT, C. A. (1971). *Flukes and Snails*. London: George Allen and Unwin Limited.

# List of worms mentioned in this book

The numbers refer to pages in the text; further references for many of the species are cited in the index. Numbers in italics refer to illustrations.

PLATYHELMINTHES (flatworms)

Turbellaria (mainly free-living)

*Fecampia erythrocephala:* body of shore crab 4

Monogenea (mainly ectoparasitic flukes)

*Amphibdella flavolineata*: gill of electric ray 5
*Calicotyle kroeri*: cloaca of ray 5
*Diclidophora denticulata*: gill of coal-fish *148*
*Diclidophora merlangi*: gill of whiting 31, 72
*Diplectanum aequans*: gill of bass 130
*Diplozoon paradoxum*: gill of freshwater fish *131*
*Entobdella soleae*: skin of common sole *6*, 31, 72
*Gyrodactylus elegans*: gill of minnow *129*
*Macrogyrodactylus polypteri*: skin of bichir (fish) *131*
*Oculotrema hippopotami*: eyelid of hippopotamus 5
*Polystoma integerrimum*: bladder of frog *6*, 31, 73

Aspidogastrea (mainly endoparasitic flukes)

*Aspidogaster limacoides*: gut of roach *6*

Digenea (mainly endoparasitic flukes)

*Alaria arisaemoides*: gut of red fox 83
*Alaria mustelae*: gut of mink 30
*Alcicornis carangis*: stomach of skipjack (fish) *12*
*Allocreadium alloneotenicum*: body of caddis fly *12*
*Apatemon gracilis minor*: gut of duck 72
*Aporocotyle macfarlani*: heart of rock fish 80
*Austrobilharzia terrigalenis*: mesenteric veins of seagull 52
*Clonorchis sinensis*: bile duct of man 178
*Coitocaecum anaspidis*: body of Tasmanian mountain shrimp 145
*Cryptocotyle lingua*: gut of sea birds 32
*Dicrocoelium dendriticum*: biliary system of sheep 53
*Diplostomum phoxini*: gut of seagull 32
*Eurytrema vulpis*: pancreatic duct of fox 72
*Fasciola hepatica*: biliary system of sheep *10*, 32, 72
*Gorgodera amplicava*: bladder of frog 73
*Haematoloechus medioplexus*: lung of frog 32, 72
*Halipegus amherstensis*: mouth of frog 48

# Index

Page numbers in italics refer to illustrations.

# THE WYKEHAM SCIENCE SERIES

|  |  |  |
|---|---|---|
| 1 | *Elementary Science of Metals* | J. W. Martin and R. A. Hull |
| 2 | †*Neutron Physics* | G. E. Bacon and G. R. Noakes |
| 3 | †*Essentials of Meteorology* | D. H. McIntosh, A. S. Thom and V. T. Saunders |
| 4 | *Nuclear Fusion* | H. R. Hulme and A. McB. Collieu |
| 5 | *Water Waves* | N. F. Barber and G. Ghey |
| 6 | *Gravity and the Earth* | A. H. Cook and V. T. Saunders |
| 7 | *Relativity and High Energy Physics* | W. G. Rosser and R. K. McCulloch |
| 8 | *The Method of Science* | R. Harré and D. G. F. Eastwood |
| 9 | †*Introduction of Polymer Science* | L. R. G. Treloar and W. F. Archenhold |
| 10 | †*The Stars: their structure and evolution* | R. J. Tayler and A. S. Everest |
| 11 | *Superconductivity* | A. W. B. Taylor and G. R. Noakes |
| 12 | *Neutrinos* | G. M. Lewis and G. A. Wheatley |
| 13 | *Crystals and X-rays* | H. S. Lipson and R. M. Lee |
| 14 | †*Biological Effects of Radiation* | J. E. Coggle and G. R. Noakes |
| 15 | *Units and Standards for Electromagnetism* | P. Vigoureux and R. A. R. Tricker |
| 16 | *The Inert Gases: Model Systems for Science* | B. L. Smith and J. P. Webb |
| 17 | *Thin Films* | K. D. Leaver, B. N. Chapman and H. T. Richards |
| 18 | *Elementary Experiments with Lasers* | G. Wright and G. E. Foxcroft |
| 19 | †*Production, Pollution, Protection* | W. B. Yapp and M. I. Smith |
| 20 | *Solid State Electronic Devices* | D. V. Morgan, M. J. Howes and J. Sutcliffe |
| 21 | *Strong Materials* | J. W. Martin and R. A. Hull |
| 22 | †*Elementary Quantum Mechanics* | Sir Nevill Mott and M. Berry |
| 23 | *The Origin of the Chemical Elements* | R. J. Tayler and A. S. Everest |
| 24 | *The Physical Properties of Glass* | D. G. Holloway and D. A. Tawney |
| 25 | *Amphibians* | J. F. D. Frazer and O. H. Frazer |
| 26 | *The Senses of Animals* | E. T. Burtt and A. Pringle |
| 27 | †*Temperature Regulation* | S. A. Richards and P. S. Fielden |
| 28 | †*Chemical Engineering in Practice* | G. Nonhebel and M. Berry |
| 29 | †*An Introduction to Electrochemical Science* | J. O'M. Bockris, N. Bonciocat, F. Gutmann and M. Berry |
| 30 | *Vertebrate Hard Tissues* | L. B. Halstead and R. Hill |
| 31 | †*The Astronomical Telescope* | B. V. Barlow and A. S. Everest |
| 32 | *Computers in Biology* | J. A. Nelder and R. D. Kime |
| 33 | *Electron Microscopy and Analysis* | P. J. Goodhew and L. E. Cartwright |
| 34 | *Introduction to Modern Microscopy* | H. N. Southworth and R. A. Hull |
| 35 | *Real Solids and Radiation* | A. E. Hughes, D. Pooley and B. Woolnough |
| 36 | *The Aerospace Environment* | T. Beer and M. D. Kucherawy |
| 37 | *The Liquid Phase* | D. H. Trevena and R. J. Cooke |
| 38 | †*From Single Cells to Plants* | E. Thomas, M. R. Davey and J. I. Williams |
| 39 | *The Control of Technology* | D. Elliott and R. Elliott |
| 40 | *Cosmic Rays* | J. G. Wilson and G. E. Perry |
| 41 | *Global Geology* | M. A. Khan and B. Matthews |
| 42 | †*Running, Walking and Jumping: The science of locomotion* | A. I. Dagg and A. James |
| 43 | †*Geology of the Moon* | J. E. Guest, R. Greeley and E. Hay |
| 44 | †*The Mass Spectrometer* | J. R. Majer and M. Berry |
| 45 | †*The Structure of Planets* | G. H. A. Cole and W. G. Watton |
| 46 | †*Images* | C. A. Taylor and G. E. Foxcroft |
| 47 | †*The Covalent Bond* | H. S. Pickering |
| 48 | †*Science with Pocket Calculators* | D. Green and J. Lewis |
| 49 | †*Galaxies: Structure and Evolution* | R. J. Tayler and A. S. Everest |
| 50 | †*Radiochemistry—Theory and Experiment* | T. A. H. Peacocke |
| 52 | †*Radioactivity in its historical and social context* | E. N. Jenkins and I. Lewis |
| 53 | †*Man-made Disasters* | B. A. Turner |

† *(Paper and Cloth Editions available.)*

4 *Sex Determination and Sexual Dimorphism in Mammals* — A. Glucksman and M. I. Smith
5 *Ultrasonics* — A. P. Cracknell and J. L. Clark
6 *Solar Energy* — J. I. B. Wilson and H. G. Brown
7 *Parasitic Worms* — D. W. T. Crompton and S. M. Joyner

# THE WYKEHAM ENGINEERING AND TECHNOLOGY SERIES

1 *Frequency Conversion* — J. Thomson, W. E. Turk and M. J. Beesley
2 *Electrical Measuring Instruments* — E. Handscombe
3 *Industrial Radiology Techniques* — R. Halmshaw
4 *Understanding and Measuring Vibrations* — R. H. Wallace
5 *Introduction to Tribology* — J. Halling and W. E. W. Smith